# Horse Nutrition and Feeding

## Second Edition

**Sarah Pilliner**
*MSc, BHSI (SM)*

**Blackwell**
Science

© 1999 Sarah Pilliner

Blackwell Science Ltd, a Blackwell
Publishing Company
Editorial Offices:
9600 Garsington Road, Oxford OX4 2DQ,
UK
  *Tel:* +44 (0)1865 776868
Blackwell Science, Inc., 350 Main Street,
Malden, MA 02148-5018, USA
  *Tel:* +1 781 388 8250
Iowa State Press, a Blackwell Publishing
Company, 2121 State Avenue, Ames, Iowa
50014-8300, USA
  *Tel:* +1 515 292 0140
Blackwell Publishing Asia Pty Ltd,
550 Swanston Street, Carlton South,
Melbourne, Victoria 3053, Australia
  *Tel:* +61 (0)3 9347 0300
Blackwell Wissenschafts Verlag,
Kurfürstendamm 57, 10707 Berlin, Germany
  *Tel:* +49 (0)30 32 79 060

First published 1992
Reprinted 1993 (twice)
Reprinted with amendments 1994
Reprinted 1995, 1996 (twice)
Second edition 1999
Reprinted 2003

Library of Congress
Cataloging-in-Publication Data
Pilliner, Sarah.
    Horse nutrition and feeding/Sarah
Pilliner. — 2nd ed.
      p.   cm.
    Includes bibliographical references
(p.   ) and index.
    ISBN 0-632-05016-0 (pbk.)
    1. Horses—Feeding and feeds.
2. Horses—Nutrition.  3. Horses—
Nutrition—Requirements.   I. Title.
SF285.5.P5   1999
636.1'084–dc21                      99-32651
                                          CIP

ISBN 0-632-05016-0

A catalogue record for this title is available
from the British Library

Set in 10/13 Palatino
by DP Photosetting, Aylesbury, Bucks
Printed and bound in India by
Replika Press Pvt, Ltd, Kundli 131028

For further information on
Blackwell Publishing, visit our website:
www.blackwellpublishing.com

# Contents

# Introduction

It takes a combination of good stable management and good training to help a horse achieve its full potential. A vital aspect of that stable management is nutrition and feeding. This book is designed to give riders, owners, trainers and students of the horse a sound knowledge of the anatomy and physiology of the horse's gut. Knowing how the gut is organised and how it works will help you understand why we feed the way we do and will highlight areas that can be improved. An understanding of the science of nutrition combined with the age-old art of feeding horses will result in happier, healthier horses, reduced feed and veterinary bills and a horse that is more likely to be able to respond to the demands that we make on it. *Horse Nutrition and Feeding* is essential reading for students planning to take British Horse Society Examinations and will provide invaluable backup to National Certificate, Advanced National Certificate, National Diploma and Higher National Diploma horse students.

The wild horse evolved over millions of years to exist on a browsing and grazing diet, living much as zebras do today: selecting the grasses and herbs it wants, grazing for short periods throughout most of the day and night and leaving its droppings behind so that the worm burden does not get too high. This system is obviously efficient – you rarely see a thin zebra. We have taken the horse and enclosed it in paddocks and stables, dramatically changing both life-style and feeding habits. Feeding time has been greatly reduced and we have introduced cereals and protein concentrates. No wonder horses are prone to colics and other problems associated with feeding. The art of feeding horses has developed over centuries to try and ensure that horses are kept as healthy as possible on this artificial regime.

The horse is a non-ruminant herbivore: in other words it exists on a diet of plants without the benefit of the complex stomachs found in ruminants such as cattle, sheep and goats. A lot of the information about horses is taken from feeding pigs; they have a simple non-ruminant gut and are thus considered to be more like horses. Obviously there are problems since pigs are not trained to racing fitness. This, plus the fact that horses are too large and expensive for much field trial work to be done on them, means that many aspects of equine nutrition are a long way behind that of other animals, and there is still a lot of mystique attached to 'good feeding'.

This book explains in simple terms the scientifically-established principles of feeding. A section on the anatomy and physiology of the horse's digestive system is followed by a look at the nutrients required by a horse to stay healthy, and the feeds available to supply those nutrients. This information is then used to develop balanced rations for different horses. Many of us keep horses at grass for much of the year and a knowledge of the basic principles of grassland management will help get the best out of our limited resources during the grassland year. These sound scientific principles are used to produce simple practical guidelines for feeding horses as diverse as orphan foals and competition horses. The horse is not a machine and even the best cared for horse may suffer dietary problems from time to time; a chapter on the more common ailments is designed to help avoid these disorders by understanding what causes them, so that good management can prevent their recurrence.

In this second edition, the chapter on the digestive system now includes a section on gut fauna, the control of digestive activity, and the transport of nutrients. The structure, function and metabolism of carbohydrate, protein and fat has been added and the information about vitamins and minerals has been updated. There are additional sections on hay alternatives and the French (INRA) Net Energy System, and the feeding of older horses and rations for working performance horses are covered. The section on worming has been updated and there is a new section on nutraceuticals, the role of feeds and feeding in maintaining the immune system and soundness.

# Chapter 1
# The Digestive System

## Introduction

The horse's ration can be classified as follows:

- There is the scientifically correct ration where all the nutrients are in acceptable ranges according to current research.
- There is the daily ration that is provided to the horse by the horse owner.
- And finally there is the ration that the horse actually consumes, which may be quite different from what the nutritionist and the horse owner intended.

Feeding horses is both a science and an art; the nutritionist and the horse owner should be able to achieve a balance between the two. The person working with the horse on a daily basis is the best person to decide if the horse is performing to his potential; this information can be used by the nutritionist to adjust the guidelines to meet the particular needs of individual horses. Being able to distinguish the individual differences and effectively adjust for them is the art of feeding.

## The digestive system

Digestion takes place in the digestive system and is the preparation of food for absorption. This includes: the mechanical forces of chewing and the muscular contractions of the gut; the chemical action of hydrochloric acid and bile; and enzymic and bacterial action. The overall function of these digestive processes is to reduce food to a state suitable for absorption. Absorption consists of the processes that result in the passage of small molecules from the gut through the gut wall and into the blood or lymph systems where they can be transported round the body and used to nourish the horse.

Animals have evolved variations in the digestive tract to allow them to utilise diets as varied as nectar in the humming bird and grass in the horse. Carnivores or meat-eating animals tend to have a diet that is relatively concentrated and highly digestible. These animals have a comparatively simple digestive tract. Omnivores and herbivores (plant-eaters) generally have a more complicated gut that has been modified to improve the utilisation of fibrous plant material. The sheep, rabbit and horse are three types of herbivore which have developed different methods of digesting a fibrous diet. The sheep is a ruminant; it has a large complex stomach followed by a long but simple small intestine, a relatively large caecum and a rather short large colon. The rabbit has a medium-sized stomach, a short and simple small intestine, a large caecum and a medium-sized large intestine. The horse has a small, simple stomach with a relatively short intestine, a large caecum and a very large hind gut. Both the rabbit and the horse have a substantial amount of hind gut fermentation.

Other large herbivores that are hind gut fermentors include the rhinoceros and the elephant and, like the horse, they eat more while digesting less of low quality fibrous feeds than most ruminants.

The digestive system consists of a tube that runs from mouth to anus (the alimentary canal) plus other organs of digestion like the liver and pancreas (Fig. 1.1). The alimentary canal can be divided up into eight major parts:

(1) mouth
(2) pharynx
(3) oesophagus or gullet
(4) stomach
(5) small intestine
(6) large intestine
(7) rectum
(8) anus

This layout is exactly the same as a dog or a human, yet we will see that there are important differences that allow the horse to survive on forage – we would not look too good on a diet of grass.

## The mouth

The horse's head is a vehicle for a great battery of grinding teeth, called molars, designed to break food down mechanically before it passes into the gut.

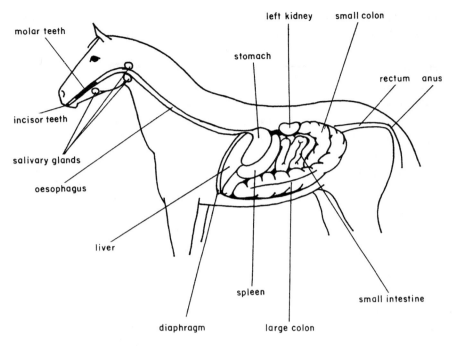

**Fig. 1.1**  The digestive system.

## The lips

The upper lip is strong, mobile and sensitive and the horse uses it to sort through the feed on offer, before manoeuvring the food between its teeth. A horse that does not like one of the ingredients of its meal is adept at sorting out and leaving the offending material. The incisor or biting teeth can bite off pieces of food in a selective fashion and, if necessary, can graze a pasture very closely.

## The tongue

The tongue then moves the food to the molar teeth for grinding, through a series of up-and-down and side-to-side chewing movements, which pulverise the food into smaller pieces suitably lubricated by saliva for swallowing. Horses have evolved as forage eaters and rely on their teeth for 'processing' this fibrous food before swallowing – all food has to be ground down to less than 2 mm in length before swallowing. Obviously this will take a lot longer for hay than for concentrates. Indeed it has been estimated that horses chew 1 kg of concentrate feed 800–1200 times but need 3000–3500 chews to get through 1 kg of hay. During this chewing saliva is produced at a rate of about 10–12 litres (3 gallons) a day. While the saliva has no digestive activity, it acts to wet and lubricate the food so that it is turned into an easily-swallowed 'porridge'. Saliva contains bicarbonate, which is alkaline and helps counteract or 'buffer' the acid produced by the horse's stomach. The horse has three salivary glands: the parotid, the sublingual and the submaxillary glands (Fig. 1.2). The other significant point regarding the mouth is that saliva is excreted only by molar pressure. People smell or see something that appeals to them and start salivating before food enters the mouth. This does not happen with horses. They only salivate when they chew food or chomp on the bit – molar pressure.

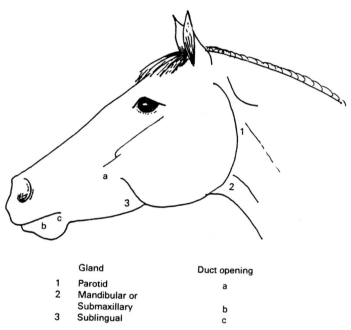

| | Gland | Duct opening |
|---|---|---|
| 1 | Parotid | a |
| 2 | Mandibular or | |
| | Submaxillary | b |
| 3 | Sublingual | c |

**Fig. 1.2**   Location of salivary glands.

## The teeth

The horse has two sets of teeth during its life:

- Temporary or milk teeth, which are smaller and whiter than the permanent teeth. From the age of two and a half years the milk teeth are gradually replaced so that by the time the horse is five years old it has a full set of
- Permanent teeth which are larger, more yellow adult teeth.

The horse has three types of tooth:

- Incisors or biting teeth in the front of the mouth (Fig. 1.3).
- Molars or grinding teeth lining each side of the jaw bone – the cheek teeth (Fig. 1.4).
- Tushes or canine teeth.

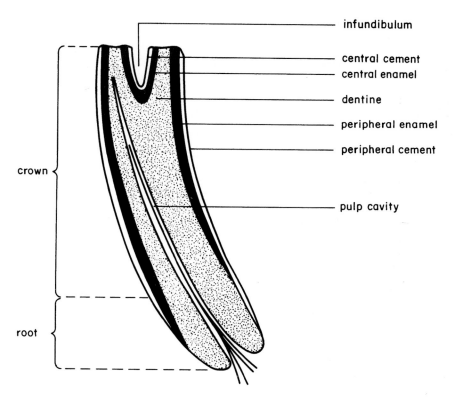

**Fig. 1.3**  The incisor tooth.

There are six incisors in each jaw: two corner, two lateral and two central incisors, which are used to age the horse. There are 12 molars to each jaw, six each side. Adult male horses (and some mares) have two tushes in each jaw, situated between the incisors and molars – thus mares have a total of 36 teeth and geldings and stallions have 40 teeth.

The horse's head is shaped so that the upper jaw is wider than the lower one; the molars overlap each other at the sides, and this allows a sideways movement of the jaw that shears the feed. As the jaw moves from side to

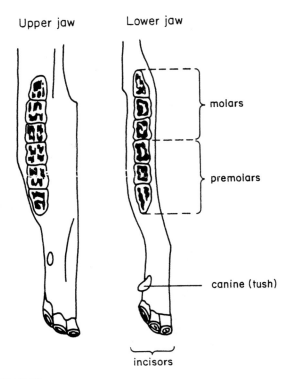

Upper jaw    Lower jaw

molars

premolars

canine (tush)

incisors

**Fig. 1.4**   The molar teeth.

side during chewing the molars grind against each other, but the lower ones do not reach the outer edge of the upper molars and the upper ones never reach the inner edge of the lower molars. The more refined the shape of the horse's head the more exaggerated this will be, resulting in sharp edges on the outside of the top molars and on the inner edge of the bottom molars (Fig. 1.5). These can cut the tongue and cheeks, making eating painful. Quidding or dropping half-chewed food out of the mouth is a sign of sharp molar teeth.

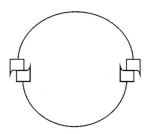

**Fig. 1.5**   Overlap of upper and lower jaws.

The vet or horse dentist can rasp or float these sharp edges and a horse's teeth should be checked twice a year and rasped if necessary.

The horse's teeth are designed to eat a fibrous diet and to cope with the vast number of chews a horse will make in its lifetime by growing continuously out from the gum to compensate for the wear caused by grinding fibrous food. The teeth are made of three different materials: cement, enamel and dentine, which have different degrees of hardness (Fig. 1.6). As the horse's teeth grind away, the enamel (which is the hardest) stands out in sharp, prominent ridges. This irregular surface is a very efficient grinding tool (Fig. 1.7).

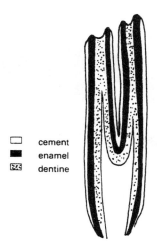

☐  cement
■  enamel
▨  dentine

**Fig. 1.6**   Section through the molar tooth.

After sufficient chewing the horse swallows a bolus of food which passes down the gullet or oesophagus to the stomach (Figs. 1.8 and 1.9). The oesophagus is a narrow muscular tube which can become blocked, leading to 'choke'.

# The stomach

## *The anatomy of the stomach*

The horse's stomach is a 'J' shaped organ lying under the diaphragm and separated from the oesophagus by a muscular ring called the cardiac sphincter. This sphincter is so powerful that it can be regarded as a one-way valve, not allowing regurgitation of gas or food. Thus the horse

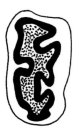

**Fig. 1.7**  Grinding surface of the molar.

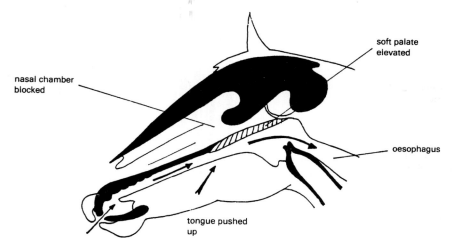

**Fig. 1.8**  Swallowing.

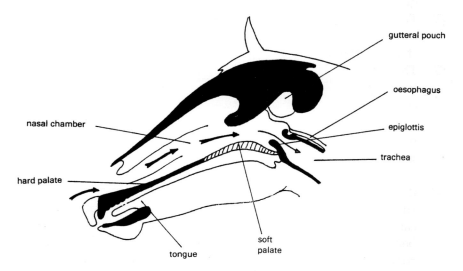

**Fig. 1.9**  Breathing.

cannot be sick, and excess gas production in the stomach cannot be relieved by burping and may result in serious colic.

The stomach can be divided into four regions: the oesophageal region or saccus caecus, the cardiac region, the fundic region and the pyloric region (Fig. 1.10).

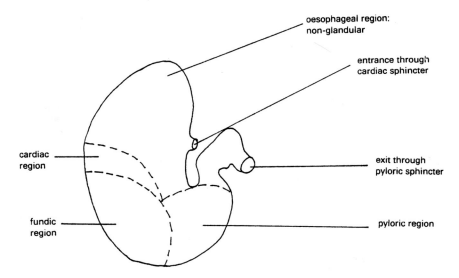

**Fig. 1.10**   Regions of the stomach.

(1)  The oesophageal region – this area does not have any digestive glands and acts as a storage area for food coming into the stomach.

(2)  The cardiac region – this area is closest to the heart and contains the cardiac glands. These glands produce mucus, possibly to protect the stomach from its own digestive juices.

(3)  The fundic region – this is the body of the stomach and contains the fundic glands (Fig. 1.11). These are the true gastric glands and are composed of three types of cells:
  • the body chief cells – produce enzymes for digestion of food;
  • the neck chief cells – secrete mucus;
  • parietal or border cells – release hydrochloric acid and an 'intrinsic factor'.

(4)  the pyloric region – contains the pyloric glands which produce a small amount of enzymes and mucus. Enzymes are catalysts; a catalyst is a substance that promotes a chemical reaction, without being changed by that reaction itself. Every living cell in the body contains catalysts or enzymes that enable the cell to carry out the complex chemical reactions that are needed to stay alive.

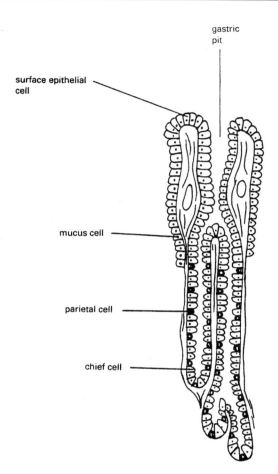

**Fig. 1.11**  Gastric gland of stomach.

The exit from the stomach to the small intestine is guarded by another strong valve known as the pyloric sphincter which controls the passage of food from the stomach.

## The practical significance of the structure of the stomach

Bear in mind that the horse is a grazing animal, evolved to be a 'trickle feeder' with a gut designed to cope with the regular intake of small quantities of fibrous food. The stabled horse, in his artificial environment, is dependent on us for his food and water, and in order to keep his digestive system working efficiently the feeding regime must mimic nature as closely as possible.

This is the reason for the Golden Rule of Good Feeding which every-body remembers best: *feed little and often* because the horse has a small stomach. As you sit on a large horse it is hard to imagine what 'small' actually means in practical terms and telling you that the stomach is ten per cent of the total gut volume does little to help. The empty stomach of a 16 hh horse is about the size of a rugby ball and can stretch to accom-modate about 13–23 litres (3–5 gallons). The 'J' shape of the stomach means that it is never more than two-thirds full, i.e. the horse's stomach will hold about 9–13 litres (2–3 gallons), about two-thirds of a standard water bucket (Fig. 1.12).

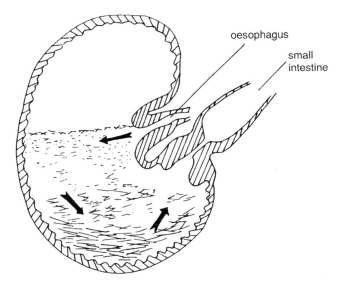

oesophagus

small
intestine

**Fig. 1.12**  Side view of opened stomach:
  (1)  Stomach never more than $\frac{2}{3}$ full
  (2)  Food lies in layers
  (3)  Food remains in stomach for 30–45 minutes
  (4)  Holds 4–5 gallons.

Allowing for the large quantity of saliva the horse produces, the best meal size is limited to just over half a bucketful – imagine a hunter's typical tea: two scoops of oats, one of nuts, half of chaff and half of sugar beet pulp – well over the half bucket. Once the horse's stomach is full, any more food eaten by the horse will push food out of the stomach before it has been treated by the digestive juices produced in the stomach. This food may ferment in the small intestine causing colic.

The small size of the stomach and the fact that the horse is a 'trickle-feeder', means that, although the stomach is rarely empty, food only stays there for a short period of time – between 30 minutes and three hours, depending on the type of feed. However the majority of a feed will have passed into the small intestine after about 45 minutes. A full stomach will also put pressure on the diaphragm, the muscular sheet which separates the lungs and the gut, preventing the horse from filling its lungs effectively – hence the rule *do not work fast for at least one hour after feeding* (Fig. 1.13). Nobody wants to go for a cross-country run straight after Sunday lunch.

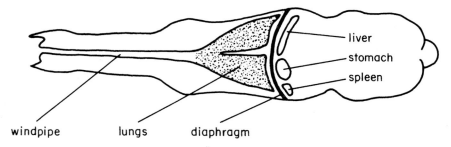

**Fig. 1.13**   Position of stomach in relation to lungs.

Another factor to consider is that during exercise blood is diverted away from the horse's gut to the muscles; food continues to pass along the gut and be digested but there is little absorption of nutrients.

Ingested food tends to form layers within the stomach. This, together with the fact that most of the water that a horse drinks follows the curvature of the 'J' shape of the stomach wall, washing over the top of the food in the stomach, means that very little of the water a horse drinks during or after a feed mixes with the stomach contents. Water also passes through the stomach wall rapidly. It is more useful to ensure that the horse has a *constant supply of fresh, clean water*, than it is to *water before feeding*.

# The small intestine

## The anatomy of the small intestine

The small intestine is a tube running from the stomach to the large intestine. It is composed of three parts: duodenum, jejunum and ileum (Fig. 1.14). In the horse the total length is about 20–27 m (65–88 feet) with a capacity of 55–70 litres (12–16 gallons). The small intestine is where most of the breakdown and absorption of the concentrate part of the

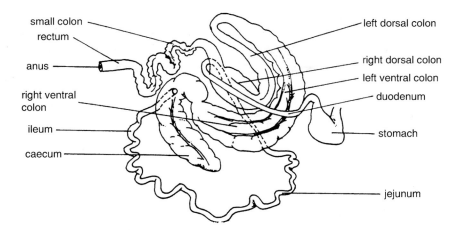

**Fig. 1.14**   The alimentary canal.

horse's diet takes place, using a similar process to that in the human, pig or dog.

- The duodenum, which is about 1 m (3 feet) long is closely attached to the stomach. It forms an S-shaped curve which contains the pancreas. The pancreatic and bile ducts enter the duodenum about 15 mm (6 inches) from the pyloric sphincter.
- The jejunum is about 20 m (65 feet) with the last 1–1.5 m (3–5 feet) being known as the ileum. The jejunum and ileum lie to the left of the horse's abdomen, between the stomach and the pelvis. The small intestine can move quite freely except at its attachment to the stomach and the caecum; it lies in numerous coils with the small colon.

There are three types of gland in the small intestine which are responsible for producing many types of digestive enzymes: intestinal glands, duodenal glands and Peyer's patches (Fig. 1.15). Intestinal glands (crypts of Lieberkuhn) and Peyer's patches are found throughout the small intestine; duodenal (Brunner's) glands are found in the first part of the small intestine.

## The large intestine

### The anatomy of the large intestine

So far the process of digestion in the horse seems little different to that in the human; however, the horse can thrive on a diet of grass, while we would look decidedly ill. What makes the horse different? The answer lies

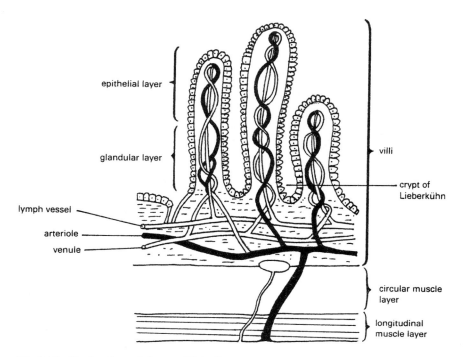

**Fig. 1.15**  Section through the small intestine.

in the horse's hind gut or large intestine, which is able to extract the energy locked up in the tough fibrous part of plants.

The horse does not have any digestive enzymes that are capable of breaking down the complex insoluble carbohydrates that make up plant cell walls. However bacteria can break down cellulose, hemicellulose and pectin by a fermentation process. The horse has a greatly-enlarged large intestine, which accommodates a vast number of micro-organisms; energy is released from the fibre in the horse's diet by fermentation of digesta by these micro-organisms. Table 1.1 shows how the horse has adapted to handle large amounts of fibrous roughage.

The large intestine extends from the ileum to the anus and is about 8 m (25 feet) long. It consists of four parts:

*The caecum*

This is a large blind-ended, comma-shaped sac situated at the end of the small intestine. The entrance to the caecum lies near the horse's right hip bone and runs forward and down 0.6–0.9 m (2–3 feet) to finish mid-way

**Table 1.1** Comparative capacity of the gastroinestinal tract of different species.

| | | Relative capacities (%) | | | |
|---|---|---|---|---|---|
| Animal | Stomach | Small intestine | Caecum | Colon and rectum | Ratio of intestinal to body length |
| Cow | 71 | 18 | 3 | 8 | 20:1 |
| Sheep | 67 | 21 | 2 | 10 | 27:1 |
| Horse | 9 | 30 | 16 | 45 | 12:1 |
| Pig | 29 | 33 | 6 | 32 | 14:1 |
| Dog | 63 | 23 | 1 | 13 | 6:1 |

along the horse's belly, lying on the floor of the abdomen. The caecum holds 25–35 litres (6–8 gallons).

### The large colon

This has a capacity of 90–110 litres (20–24 gallons) and a length of 3–4 m (10–13 feet). In order to fit into the horse's abdomen the large colon has to fold into four regions (Fig. 1.16). The first part, the right ventral colon, runs forward from the top of the caecum, lying against the horse's right flank until it reaches the sternal flexure. Here the diameter of the colon narrows and it turns back on itself to continue backwards as the left ventral colon, running on the left side of the horse to the pelvic region. The colon then turns again at the pelvic flexure, the diameter reducing to as little as 9 cm (2.5 inches), before it expands rapidly to continue towards the diaphragm as the left dorsal colon. The colon makes a final turn at the diaphragmatic flexure and the right dorsal colon runs backwards, narrowing to become the small colon. The large intestine is only held in place in the abdomen by its bulk; if the gut is too empty problems may arise.

The points where the colon narrows and turns are vulnerable to blockage. If for any reason, the passage of digesta through the colon is slowed down, obstruction and hence colic may occur; think of the tail-back that closing off one lane of the motorway can cause. Most digesta reaches the caecum three hours after a meal and remains in the large intestine for 36–48 hours.

### The small colon

This is 3–4 m (10–13 feet) long but is narrower than the large colon and only has a capacity of 9–70 litres (2–16 gallons). The small colon lies

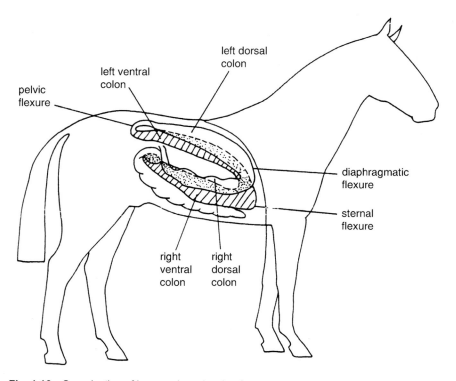

**Fig. 1.16**  Organisation of large, colon, showing flexures.

intermingled with the jejunum; it is fairly free to move and this can lead to abdominal crises such as 'twisted gut'.

*The rectum*

This is a short, relatively straight tube connecting the small colon to the anus and acting as a storage area for faeces.

## The physiology of digestion

The digestive processes that take place in the horse are different from other grass-eaters such as the cow, which is a ruminant. In the horse easily-digested food material is first hydrolysed by the action of digestive enzymes; only insoluble material reaches the large intestine for bacterial fermentation. This insoluble material is mainly cellulose. In the wild the horse is a trickle feeder, eating a mainly fibrous diet, and this arrangement is very efficient. In an all-hay diet over 70 per cent of the horse's energy is derived from hind gut digestion. Stabled horses tend to be given three feeds a day; this food passes rapidly through the gut and there is insufficient time for all the soluble material to be completely digested by the enzymes in the small intestine. Remaining soluble material passes into the caecum, which is not only wasteful but can cause severe digestive upset (this will be discussed in detail later). This is a strong argument for spreading the horse's feed over the day – *feed little and often*.

## Digestion in the stomach

In fact there is relatively little digestion of food in the stomach, but the acid stomach secretions physically break down the feed and kill any bacteria that may have been ingested.

Arrival of the feed in the stomach stimulates the release of gastric juices from the fundic glands, containing enzymes and acid. The enzymes are pepsin and gastric lipase:

- Pepsin is a protein-digesting enzyme which is secreted in the form of pepsinogen. Pepsinogen is activated to pepsin by acid. Pepsin does not break down protein completely, but results in intermediate products called proteoses and peptones.
- Gastric lipase only occurs in small amounts and is involved in the reduction of fat to fatty acids and glycerol; its action in the stomach is minimal.
- The hydrochloric acid produced by the parietal cells is one of the most important constituents of gastric juice; it activates pepsin and acts as an antiseptic solution for the stomach.

The action of chewing causes large amounts of saliva to be produced. Saliva is alkaline and, when swallowed along with the food, helps to counteract the acidic environment in the stomach. The result is a marked variation in the acidity of the food in different regions of the stomach. Near the entrance the material is neutral, in the fundic region it is slightly acidic and in the pyloric region it is very acid. This highly acid area stimulates pepsin activation and protein digestion. The amount of protein digestion is limited by the small size of the stomach and the short period of time that the food is actually in the stomach.

A certain amount of fermentation of material takes place in the less acidic oesophageal and fundic regions of the stomach, resulting in lactic acid, which makes little nutritional contribution.

## Digestion in the small intestine

Digestion in the stomach is acid but the enzymes in the small intestine need alkaline conditions. This alkalinity is mainly produced by pancreatic juice from the pancreas and bile from the liver. The partially digested food from the stomach, now called chyme, is acted on by enzymes to produce materials that can be absorbed by the body.

### The pancreas

The pancreas has a dual purpose: one is the control of blood sugar levels and glucose metabolism via the hormone insulin, the other is the production of enzyme-containing pancreatic juice. Although the production of pancreatic juice is continuous, the presence of food in the stomach increases the rate of production by four to five times – up to 20 litres (4.5 gallons) over 24 hours.

### Bile

Bile from the liver enters the small intestine via the bile duct. Unlike the human the horse does not have a gall bladder for the storage of bile; instead bile trickles continuously into the duodenum. This serves to remind us once again that the horse evolved as a trickle feeder, needing frequent, small feeds. Bile contains salts of bile acids (glycocholates and taurocholates) which are important in providing an alkaline pH in the small intestine and in preparing fats for absorption by the formation of micelles in the lumen of the intestine; micelles are aggregates of molecules of lipids and bile acids. The bile salts are absorbed in the small intestine and returned to the liver. Bile pigments, including bilirubin and biliverdin, are responsible for the characteristic colour of bile and most of the colour in faeces and urine. These pigments are waste products of the breakdown of blood pigment, haemoglobin, in the liver. Bile is also a way of excreting many metallic elements and inactivated hormones.

Ingesta is moved along the intestine and mixed with digestive secretions by movements of the intestine. There are three types of movement:

- Propulsive movements designed to push the ingesta from mouth to anus, known as peristalsis.
- Absorptive movements designed to mix the ingesta with the digestive juices and to bring ingesta into contact with the intestine wall for absorption of nutrients.
- Control movements which start and stop peristalsis.

## The digestive enzymes

Enzymes help reduce complex food materials into simple substances which can be absorbed. Essentially digestive enzymes fall into three major categories, which are specific for a type of nutrient:

*Protein-digesting enzymes (proteases)*

- Pepsin
- Trypsin
- Chymotrypsin
- Carboxypeptidase
- Erepsin
- Aminopeptidase
- Polynucleotidase
- Nucleotidase
- Nucleosidase

*Carbohydrate-digesting enzymes (amylases)*

- Pancreatic amylase
- Sucrase
- Maltase
- Lactase

*Fat-digesting enzymes (lipases)*

- Gastric lipase
- Pancreatic lipase
- Intestinal lipase
- Phospholipase

The rate of passage of material through the small intestine is quite rapid and food particles will pass through into the caecum in just over an hour. Non-fibrous, soluble feeds will be substantially digested in this short period of time through the action of the digestive enzymes.

### Fat digestion

Fat digestion is the result of the emulsifying effect of bile salts and the enzymic action of pancreatic and intestinal lipases. Pancreatic lipase hydrolyses fatty acids to produce two free fatty acids and a 2-mono-

**Table 1.2**  Summary of enzyme digestion in the horse.

| Origin | Enzyme | Substrate | End product |
|---|---|---|---|
| *Mouth* | | | |
|   salivary glands | Salivary amylase | Activity minimal in horses | |
| *Stomach* | | | |
|   body chief cells | Pepsin | Proteins | Proteoses and peptones |
|   fundic neck chief cells | Gastric lipase | Fats | Fatty acid and glycerol |
| *Pancreas* | Trypsin | Proteins, proteoses, peptones, polypeptides | Peptones, peptides amino acids. Also activates chymotrypsin. |
| | Chymotrypsin | As for trypsin | As for trypsin |
| | Pancreatic amylase | Starch and dextrins | Dextrins, maltose |
| | Pancreatic amylase | Fats | Fatty acids, glycerol |
| | Carboxypeptidase | Peptides with a free carboxyl | Amino acids |
| *Small intestine* | | | |
|   crypts of Leiberkühn | Erepsin | Peptides, proteoses, peptones | Amino acids |
| | Aminopeptidases | Peptides | Amino acids |
| | Sucrase | Sucrose | Glucose, fructose |
| | Lactase | Lactose | Glucose, galactose |
| | Maltase | Maltose | Glucose |
| | Nucleotidase | Mononucleotides | Nucleosides |
| | Nucleosidase | Nucleosides | Purine and pyrimidine bases, pentoses |
| | Enterokinase (activates Trypsin) | Trypsinogen | Trypsin |

glyceride. The bile salts and hydrolysed fats form micelles, which increases the surface area of the fat droplets by a factor of up to 10 000. The micelles are absorbed by the intestinal epithelium into the lymph system, which empties into the vena cava. Horses can digest fat very effectively, even though traditional horse diets are low in fat. The composition of the horse's body fat is affected by the type of fat in the diet; in this respect the horse resembles the human being rather than the cow.

*Protein digestion*

In contrast to the limited breakdown of protein in the stomach, protein digestion in the small intestine is extensive. Proteins are eventually broken down to the simple building blocks called amino acids, which are absorbed across the gut wall into the blood stream. The protein in insoluble fibrous feeds is not easily digested in the small intestine; it is mainly the protein from the concentrate part of the ration which is digested here.

## Carbohydrate digestion

The water-soluble carbohydrates such as sugars and cereal starches are broken down in the small intestine. The stabled horse on a high con-centrate diet will be receiving a large proportion of its dietary energy as starch, making the efficiency of small intestine digestion significant. Horses are not well adapted to digest starch; they evolved to eat grass, which has only a low starch content. Starch is chemically complex, made of many glucose molecules bonded together. It can be a problem for a horse to break down these bonds in the short time that the material is in the small intestine. The cooked starch found in extruded and micronised feeds is much easier for the horse to deal with. If the horse cannot digest all the starch in the small intestine and it passes through to the large intestine, it may be the forerunner of problems such as laminitis and colic.

## Digestion in the large intestine

Throughout the large intestine water is absorbed from the digesta, so that by the time it reaches the rectum it has a firm consistency. The main function of the caecum and large colon is to provide a suitable environ-ment to house millions of micro-organisms – there are ten times more bacteria in the horse's gut than there are cells in its body and more than half the dry weight of the faeces is actually bacteria.

Animals do not produce enzymes that hydrolyse complex carbohy-drates such as xylan, cellulose and hemicellulose; any hydrolysis of these compounds is due to microbial activity. The micro-organisms ferment insoluble carbohydrate to produce volatile fatty acids (VFA), principally acetic, proprionic and butyric acids. These are absorbed into the horse's bloodstream and used as a source of energy, allowing the horse to thrive on its natural forage diet. The numbers and types of bacteria in the gut are dependent on the type of ration being fed. It is important to maintain a consistent diet so that the population of bacteria is in a steady state. Sudden changes upset the microbial population leading to digestive upsets: *make all dietary changes gradually.*

**Table 1.3**  Summary of digestion in the horse.

| | Secretion | Digestion products | Absorbed | Material passed on |
|---|---|---|---|---|
| Stomach | Hydrochloric acid<br>Unknown intrinsic factor<br>Mucus | Lactic acid | Minimal | All ingesta and gastric secretions |
| Small intestine | Sodium bicarbonate<br>Pancreatic enzymes<br>Bile<br>Mucus | Amino acids<br>Glucose and other simple sugars<br>Triglycerides and fatty acids | Amino acids<br>Simple sugars<br>Fatty acids<br>Vitamins<br>Calcium, magnesium, potassium, chloride | Fibre, water |
| Caecum | Water | Volatile fatty acids<br>B vitamins<br>Microbial protein | Volatile fatty acids<br>Vitamins*<br>Amino acids* | Fibre |
| Large colon | | VFAs<br>B vitamins | VFAs<br>Thiamin<br>Amino acids<br>Water | Indigestible components |

* The amounts absorbed are questionable

## Microbial numbers

In the fundic region of the stomach, there are from $10^8$–$10^9$ bacteria/g. As the pH is about 5.4 the bacteria are those which can withstand moderate acidity, including lactobacilli and streptococci . The jejunum and ileum of the small intestine houses $10^8$–$10^9$ bacteria/g, mainly anaerobic Gram-positive bacteria; the cereal content of the horse's diet will influence the proportion of each type of bacteria.

The bacteria of the caecum and colon number about $0.5 \times 10^9$–$5 \times 10^9$/g and have an optimum pH of 5–6. The bacterial population is highest in the caecum and ventral colon with about seven times more cellulose-digesting bacteria than in the terminal colon.

The numbers of specific micro-organisms fluctuates dramatically in the meal-fed domesticated horse, with 100-fold changes during 24 hours. This reflects the changes in the availability of nutrients and changes in pH. Changing the ratio of hay to concentrates that the horse receives influences;

- numbers of micro-organisims
- types of micro-organisms.

Frequency of feeding has an effect on metabolic and digestive disorders which relates directly to the effect of diet and feeding practice on the microbial population. Horses are not designed to be given infrequent meals or to eat cereals.

Bacteria become adapted to a specific substrate; thus caecal bacteria from a horse on a cereal diet are less efficient at digesting hay and if a sudden change is made to a hay diet, impaction may occur. Bacteria from a horse on a hay ration are not as efficient at digesting cereals and an abrupt change to a cereal diet may result in colic, laminitis or filled legs.

A change in the ratio of starch to fibre in the diet leads to a change in the proportions of VFA yielded, with acetate and butyrate being the major products of fibre digestion. The proportion of propionate and lactate increases as the starch levels of the diet increase. The optimum pH for microbial activity is 6.5 and this pH also promotes VFA absorption into the bloodstream. Microbial activity also produces gases, mainly carbon dioxide and methane. These gases can cause problems, such as colic, if the rate of production exceeds the rate of disposal.

### Protozoa

Protozoa number about $0.5 \times 10^5 - 1.5 \times 10^5/g$. There are far fewer protozoa than bacteria and their contribution to metabolism is less, but as they are much bigger they contribute about the same total mass. Seventy-two species of protozoa have been found in the horse's large intestine.

There is a delicate balance between the lactic acid-producing bacteria and those that convert the lactic acid into VFAs. Any soluble carbohydrate arriving in the caecum is rapidly broken down by Lactobacilli to give lactic acid; if the other bacteria cannot rapidly reduce the lactic acid to harmless VFAs, the acid will build up and cause serious metabolic problems.

The bacteria themselves consist of a high percentage of protein. The essential amino acids in this protein are not very available to the horse (unlike the cow), because the large intestine does not contain the necessary protein-digesting enzymes. This means that horses, particularly youngstock, need good quality protein. The bacteria also provide the horse with some of the B vitamins needed for health.

As the competition horse is fed more concentrates, more emphasis is placed on digestion in the small intestine and there are fewer micro-organisms in the hind gut: this 'grain atrophy' has implications which will be discussed later.

## Control of digestive activity

The digestive system is controlled by a combination of nerve stimulation and inhibition and a number of specific hormones. The nerve supply of the oesophagus, stomach, small intestine and proximal part of the large intestine is via the vagus nerve. The sacral segment of the spinal cord supplies the distal portion of the colon, rectum and the internal anal sphincter. Control is also through gastrointestinal peptide hormones and hormone-like peptides which stimulate and reduce secretion, motility and absorption. These neural and endocrine controls result in a coordinated sequence of action; orderly muscle action serves to mix and transport digesta through the gut while the secretions necessary for the digestion and absorption of nutrients are released. Adrenal and para-thyroid hormones also have an effect while other hormones such as insulin and glucagon from the pancreas affect nutrient utilisation.

## Transport of nutrients

Most of the absorption of nutrients takes place in the duodenum and jejunum and, to a lesser extent, the ileum and large intestine. As the passage of ingesta from mouth to caecum takes only a couple of hours in the horse, there is limited opportunity for processing and absorbing nutrients. The amount of absorption is increased if the surface area of the intestine is increased. For example, if the human intestine was a simple cylinder, the surface area would be about $3300\,cm^2$; however, the actual surface area is about 2 million $cm^2$. This increase is brought about by folds, villi and microvilli.

The passage of individual nutrients from the lumen of the intestine, through the intestinal epithelial cell and into the blood or lymph may occur in several ways:

- passive diffusion
- active transport
- pinocytosis.

Pinocytosis involves the particle being engulfed in a similar manner to the way an amoeba surrounds its food. This occurs in new-born foals to allow the absorption of large immune globulin molecules.

Active transport or diffusion both involve:

- penetration of the microvillus and of the plasma membrane, which encapsulates the epithelial cell
- migration through the cell
- possible metabolism within the cell
- extrusion from the cell
- passage through the basement membrane
- penetration through the vascular or lymphatic epithelium into the blood or lymph.

If the nutrient enters the blood capillaries, it is carried by the portal vein to the liver. The liver acts as a central organ in metabolism with many complex and vital reactions taking place.

# Chapter 2
# The Necessary Nutrients

To remain healthy and to do the work we demand, the horse requires a balance of over 40 nutrients. These fall into six categories:

(1)  carbohydrate
(2)  protein
(3)  fat

(4)  minerals
(5)  vitamins
(6)  water.

## Carbohydrate

Carbohydrates are the major components in plant tissues; they make up about 70 per cent of the dry matter of most forages and can comprise up to 85 per cent of cereal grains. The chloroplasts in plant leaves synthesise carbohydrate via a process called photosynthesis, using energy from the sun, carbon dioxide and water and releasing oxygen. Animals also contain carbohydrates, mainly in the form of glucose and glycogen.

All carbohydrates are characterised by being made up of the elements carbon, hydrogen and oxygen, with the hydrogen and oxygen usually present in the 2:1 ratio found in water. This gives rise to the name carbohydrate: carbo- (carbon) hydrate (water). Carbohydrates can be classified on the basis of the number of carbon atoms per molecule of carbohydrate and the number of molecules of sugar in the compound.

Carbohydrates provide the energy needed for all cell processes and basic functions such as breathing and the beating of the heart. They also provide energy for muscle contraction, and consequently performance horses need high levels of carbohydrate in their diet. If carbohydrates are fed in excess, any energy not burned up is stored as fat – as those of us too fond of bread, cakes and potatoes know only too well.

### Sugars and starch

Sugars and starch are soluble carbohydrates; they are built up of molecules of the simple sugar, glucose. Before they can be absorbed across the wall of the gut they are broken down by digestive enzymes to glucose, which is used by the body for basic cell function – essentially keeping the horse alive. Glucose is a very important energy source, and is the preferred source of energy for most body tissues, and the only type of energy that can be used by red blood cells and the medulla of the kidney. It is important for the horse to maintain a blood-glucose concentration within certain defined limits. Both sugars and starches are found in large quantities in the horse's concentrate ration. They are comparatively easily digested by enzyme activity in the small intestine, providing a fairly instant supply of energy.

### Monosaccharides

The most simple carbohydrates are simple sugars containing only one molecule of sugar and include:

Pentoses ($C_5H_{10}O_5$)

- arabinose
- xylose
- ribose.

Hexoses ($C_6H_{12}O_6$)

- glucose
- fructose
- galactose
- mannose.

Glucose is the main fuel for cells, providing the energy for normal life processes.

### Disaccharides

Disaccharides contain two molecules of sugar:

- sucrose        glucose + fructose
- maltose        glucose + glucose
- lactose        glucose + galactose
- cellobiose     glucose + glucose

Sucrose is the sugar found in sugar cane and sugar beet and the form of sugar which we most commonly use. Lactose is milk sugar and cellobiose is found in the fibrous portion of plants.

### Trisaccharides

Trisaccharides contain three molecules of sugar:

- raffinose          glucose + fructose + galactose

Raffinose is found in cottonseed, some varieties of eucalyptus and sugar beet.

### Polysaccharides

Polysaccharides are long chains of sugar molecules:

- starch              glucose              grains, seeds, tubers
- cellulose           glucose              plant cell walls
- glycogen            glucose              liver, muscle
- hemicellulose       hexoses + pentoses   fibrous plants

Starch is the storage form of sugar in plants, with particularly high levels in cereal grains. The horse stores sugar as glycogen in the liver and muscles. Both starch and glycogen are made up of glucose molecules coiled into a helical shape but the glycogen chain is more branched than that of starch. Many polysaccharides have a structural function and provide strength and rigidity; for example, cellulose forms the fundamental structure of all plant cell walls and is more commonly known as fibre.

### Cellulose

A large part of the horse's carbohydrate intake is made up of cellulose, the complex structural part of plants. Cellulose is a highly complicated substance, contributing strength to plant cell walls, enabling grasses to stand upright. Cellulose and other structural carbohydrates, such as hemicellulose and pectin, are insoluble carbohydrates and resist enzyme breakdown. Instead they are fermented by the bacteria of the hind gut to yield volatile fatty acids (VFAs), which can be used by the horse to produce energy.

Excess carbohydrate in the ration causes obesity, while a deficiency results in the horse breaking down body reserves to supply necessary energy. The horse will lose condition and eventually become emaciated.

Like starch and glycogen, cellulose is also made up of glucose molecules but these are linked together to form long rods with no branches. Hemicelluloses contain many different sugar molecules forming mixed polysaccharides which are abundant in pasture and hence conserved forages.

### Lignin

Lignin is not a carbohydrate but is a mixture of polymers of phenolic acid and is closely associated with this group; it gives mechanical strength to plants, increasing as the plant ages. Lignin is indigestible and results in grass becoming less digestible as it matures; wood, straw, hay and mature pasture are all high in lignin.

## Metabolism

Only monosaccharides can be absorbed from the gut, thus di-, tri- and polysaccharides must be hydrolysed by digestive enzymes or micro-organisms. Unlike the glucose links in starch and glycogen those in cellulose cannot be broken down by the enzymes produced by the horse's gut. This means that all herbivores, including the horse need to utilise micro-organisms which produce the enzyme cellulase in order to digest cellulose. The end products of this digestion are volatile fatty acids.

Conversion of some monosaccharides to glucose occurs in the intestinal mucosal cells during absorption, the remainder may be converted to glucose in the liver. The horse stores little energy as carbohydrate but some glucose is converted to glycogen for storage in the liver and muscle tissues. The level of blood glucose is maintained within a narrow range by conversion of circulating blood glucose to glycogen and by reconversion to glucose when blood sugar levels fall. Blood glucose rises after a meal but returns to normal levels within a short time; this homeostasis is under endocrine control, with the hormones insulin and glucagon from the pancreas playing a vital role.

### Energy production

In order for a cell to function it has to be able to extract and use the chemical energy within glucose; when glucose is broken down, carbon dioxide, water and energy are released. The cell can capture some of this energy by transferring it to an energy carrier molecule, for example, adenosine triphosphate (ATP). This molecule consists of an adenosine body with three phosphate attachments. When one of the phosphates is lost to form adenosine diphosphate (ADP), energy is released and can be used to power the cell. This reaction takes place in the mitochondria of the cell.

### Glycolysis

Glycogen consists of molecules of glucose polymerised to form a complex polysaccharide; in glycolysis, successive molecules of glucose in the polymer chain are split off the main body by a process called phosphorylation. The hormones glucagon and adrenalin both activate the enzyme, phosphorylase, which allows the process to take place.

The resulting glucose molecules are phosphorylated, in other words they each have a phosphate group attached to them. The phosphorylated glucose can either continue down the glycolytic pathway or, if the phosphate group is removed, the glucose can pass out of the cell and be transported in the blood to other cells which need energy.

Glycolysis is known as anaerobic respiration and does not require the presence of oxygen to take place. However, during the glycolysis of glucose to pyruvic acid only two ATP molecules are produced and a lot of energy is lost as heat, making this reaction only 25 per cent effective. In addition, in the absence of oxygen, the pyruvic acid is converted to lactic acid which can accumulate in the muscle cells contributing to fatigue. In order for the pyruvic acid to be converted to carbon dioxide and water, respiratory oxygen is needed.

### The Krebs or tricarboxylic (TCA) cycle

The conversion of pyruvic acid to carbon dioxide and water releases hydrogen atoms which are oxidised, through oxidative phosphorylation, to produce ATP. The complete oxidation of one molecule of glucose to carbon dioxide and water results in 38 units of ATP. This process requires oxygen and is known as aerobic respiration, and is more efficient than anaerobic respiration, although it also results in substantial heat loss.

## Protein

Proteins are essential organic constituents of all living organisms, all cells contain proteins and they are found in high concentration in muscle tissue. All cells make proteins during their life cycle and without protein manufacture, life could not exist. The protein requirement is highest for young growing animals and declines as the animal matures so that the adult requires only a maintenance level. Pregnancy and lactation increase the protein requirement.

Proteins vary in chemical composition, physical properties and biological function. However, they are all made up of simple building blocks called amino acids. The essential components of an amino acid are a carboxyl group and an amino group ($NH_2$) on the C atom next to the carboxyl group. There are over 200 amino acids but only 20 are found in most proteins and up to 10 are required in the diet because tissue synthesis is unable to meet demand. The synthesis of protein from amino acids occurs by linking amino acids to form long chains. The length of the chain and the order of the amino acids determines the properties of the protein. The link between the amino acids is called a peptide bond. Most proteins contain 350–5000 amino acid residues. The 20 amino acids can also be arranged in nearly any sequence. This enormous diversity of structure results in proteins as different as hair, leather, enzymes and meat.

All proteins can be classified into three main groups:

- globular proteins such as albumins and globulins
- fibrous proteins such as collagens and keratins
- conjugated proteins which contain non-protein compounds.

Proteins have many different functions including:

- cell membranes
- muscle tissue
- skin, hair and hooves
- blood plasma proteins
- enzymes
- hormones
- immune antibodies.

## Protein metabolism

During digestion proteins are hydrolysed to amino acids and absorbed across the wall of the small intestine into the portal circulation which takes them to the liver. The nutritive value of a protein in the diet depends not only on its digestibility and absorbability but also on the utilisation of its component amino acids after absorption. In the liver the amino acids may be metabolised or transferred directly into the blood stream. The processing reactions include:

- synthesis of body protein
- synthesis of enzymes and hormones
- conversion of ammonia into urea
- gluconeogenesis – the conversion of protein to carbohydrate for energy. This is normally a low-level activity but during disease and starvation may be a major source of energy, resulting in the wastage of muscle.

## Protein deficiency

Signs of protein deficiency include anorexia, reduced growth rate, and reduced efficiency of feed utilisation. Deficiencies of individual essential amino acids generally produce these signs because lack of a single amino acid prevents protein accretion. Most individual feed stuffs are inadequate in one or more amino acids for growing animals; for example, maize is deficient in lysine, but this can be balanced with soyabean meal which is rich in lysine. The horse's diet must meet both the total protein needs and the requirement for individual amino acids.

## Protein quality

Horses can make ten amino acids in the body; however the rest cannot be synthesised at all or cannot be made fast enough to meet the horse's protein requirement. Plants and many micro-organisms can synthesise all the amino acids. This means that horses have to get the amino acid that they cannot make from the plants in their diet. Microbial protein in the horse's large intestine is probably not significant as a source of amino acids.

The amino acids that cannot be made by the horse are called essential amino acids. Proteins that contain a high level of these essential amino acids are said to have a high biological value and are good quality proteins which horses need in their diet.

If one of the essential amino acids is only present in the diet in small amounts, it will upset the balance and limit the use of the other amino acids, leading to an apparent protein deficiency. A horse fed a traditional ration of hay, oats and bran, will have a low level of the essential amino acid lysine. This will limit the horse's ability to use the rest of the protein

**Table 2.1**  Amino acids.

| Essential amino acids | Non-essential amino acids |
|---|---|
| Lysine | Glycine |
| Methionine | Glutamic acid |
| Threonine | Cysteine |
| Phenylalanine | Citrulline |
| Isoleucine | Di-iodotyrosine |
| Histidine | Aspartic acid |
| Valine | Serine |
| Tryptophan | Hydroxyproline |
| Leucine | Cystine |
| | Thyroxine |
| | Alanine |
| | Proline |
| | Tyrosine |
| | Hydroxylisine |

in the diet. Lysine is thus known as the limiting amino acid in that ration.

Protein is used in the body for the maintenance of healthy tissue, growth and development, milk production and pregnancy. Tissue proteins are broken down and resynthesised during normal maintenance of all horses. This process is not fully efficient so there is a continual need for protein in the diet to make good the loss. Protein is also lost from the body in secretions, in the sloughing off of the tissue lining the gut, respiratory tract and urinary tract, and the loss of hair. Protein makes up a large percentage of muscle tissue, and thus growth and development, milk production and pregnancy have a much higher protein requirement.

# Fat

Fats or lipids are organic compounds which have important biochemical and physiological functions:

- supply energy
- source of essential fatty acids
- carrier of fat-soluble vitamins
- integral constituent of cell membranes.

Fats or lipids occur in several forms:

- simple lipids, e.g. triglycerides – fats and oils which are esters of fatty acids with glycerol
- compound lipids, e.g. phospholipids – containing substances such as phosphorus, carbohydrates or proteins
- sterols, e.g. cholesterol – complex lipids.

The most important constituents, from a nutritional point are fatty acids, glycerol, triglycerides and phospholipids. Triglycerides are the main storage form of energy in the horse's body.

## Fatty acids

Triglycerides and phospholipids contain fatty acids characterised by a long chain of carbon atoms linked to hydrogen atoms. The fewer hydrogen atoms in the chain, the less saturated and more fluid the fatty acids will be.

## Glycerol

Glycerol is the alcohol component of triglycerides.

## Triglycerides

Triglycerides are esters of glycerol and fatty acids. An ester is formed by the reaction of an alcohol with an organic acid. The chain length and degree of unsaturation of the fatty acids determine the physical and chemical properties of the triglyceride. Simple triglycerides with fewer than ten carbons are usually liquid at room temperature.

## Essential fatty acids

Linoleic, arachidonic and linolenic acid are not produced in sufficient quantities by the horse and must be supplied in the diet. These fatty acids are an integral part of cell membranes and also have a role in the production of prostaglandins. The importance of these and other fatty acids such as omega-3 fatty acids in the diet is not fully understood.

## Fat digestion

During digestion fats are emulsified and then hydrolysed to glycerol and fatty acids which pass across the wall of the small intestine to be resynthesised into triglycerides, before passing into the lacteals. The fat droplets are transported to the bloodstream by the lymphatic system. Once in the blood the majority of the absorbed fat is hydrolysed to fatty acids and glycerol.

### Triglyceride metabolism

All tissues of the body store triglycerides, with adipose tissue (fat depots) being the most important storage sites. Adipose tissue can synthesise fat from carbohydrate and is capable of the oxidation of fatty acids. Energy intake in excess of requirements results in storage of triglycerides (fattening) and energy intake less than that required results in loss of triglycerides.

The liver plays a major role in the breakdown of triglycerides for energy production; it is also able to form specialised fatty acids. In the breakdown of lipids, triglycerides in the fat depots are first hydrolysed to fatty acids and glycerol. The glycerol then passes through the phosphogluconate pathway to release energy. The fatty acids are transported via the blood to various body tissues to be used as an oxidative energy source. Oxidation takes place in the mitochondria of the cells where fatty acids are converted into acetyl-CoA, which enters the Krebs cycle. Fat is very energy dense and produces more energy than the breakdown of carbohydrate.

Horse diets rarely contain more than about 4 per cent of fat. Compare this with over 50 per cent in many human diets. Fat is a highly concentrated source of energy and horses are able to digest fat quite efficiently. The addition of edible fat to the horse's diet can be useful, particularly for the endurance horse. Adding a cup of oil to each of a horse's three feeds (0.3 litres) is equivalent in energy terms to feeding 1 kg of oats.

## Minerals and vitamins

One of the aims of providing an optimal diet for the horse is to ensure that he receives adequate vitamins and minerals in the ration. Vitamins and minerals are essential for body function and they operate at all levels from energy production to hoof growth. Deficiencies and toxicities of minerals and vitamins may show themselves clinically either extremely rapidly or over a long period of time. Theoretically there are five grades for the supply of an element in the horse's diet:

- Deficient supply, characterised by clinical symptoms; in other words, the horse actually looks ill.
- Suboptimal supply; there are biochemical changes in the horse's metabolism but there are no clinical symptoms. The horse's body is not functioning properly but he does not appear to be ill. This is a difficult situation to identify; the horse is not fully healthy yet he shows no signs of being unwell. This is probably why mineral and vitamin supplementation has become full of mystery and mis-understanding, with owners almost frightened not to feed a supplement.
- Optimal supply; this ensures full health and performance capacity.
- Subtoxic supply; this is characterised by biochemical changes in the horse's metabolism and body functions but these are not associated with clinical symptoms.
- Toxic intake; the level is such that clinical symptoms are seen.

Just to complicate matters further, many minerals and vitamins play multiple roles or alternatively have very specific functions. Some elements may interfere with the absorption and uptake of other elements. Overfeeding one substance may create an artifical deficiency of another, which means that there are actually adequate amounts in the diet which the horse is unable to utilise, because of the very high levels of the interfering element. For example, feeding high levels of phosphorus can lead to a calcium deficiency; even though it would appear that calcium levels were adequate, phosphorus effectively 'holds on to' the calcium and the horse's body cannot use it. This mineral interaction is an important factor in horse nutrition, an imbalance of minerals being just as important as an actual deficiency in many nutritional disorders.

Horse owners must not only be aware of the critical role that minerals and vitamins play in horse nutrition. They must also be alert to the dangers of over-supplementation. Not only will the absorption of some minerals and vitamins be impeded but overdosing with some minerals, for example copper (Cu), will eventually produce toxic symptoms – *you will poison your horse.* Other elements that are potentially poisonous are selenium (Se) and molybdenum (Mo). Supplementation of any diet should be done with great care and the indiscriminate use of trace elements must be avoided.

# Minerals

## The roles of the essential minerals

The term *essential* is only used for those mineral elements that have been proved to have a role in the horse's metabolic processes. The classification of these minerals into either major or trace elements is dependent on the concentration in the body. Normally trace elements are present in a concentration below 50 milligrams per kilogram (mg/kg).

## The major minerals

### Calcium (Ca) and phosphorus (P)

Calcium and phosphorus can be considered together as their functions are very closely related. They are the main elements of the apatite crystal which provides strength and stability to the skeleton. Bone acts as a reservoir of both calcium and phosphorus, with the minerals being removed and deposited as necessary, allowing the bone to be remodelled during growth and development and making up any shortfall in the diet. Calcium is also involved in blood coagulation, lactation, and nerve and muscle function; it also acts as an enzyme activator and inhibitor. Bone has a Ca:P ratio of 2:1 but the ratio in the whole body is about 1.7:1. Owing to its vital role, blood levels of calcium are kept within closely defined limits.

Diets high in wheat bran and cereals are high in phosphorus and low in calcium and may cause calcium deficiency. A lack of calcium and phosphorus in the diet of growing foals delays the closure of the epiphyseal plates of the long bones and is associated with Developmental Orthopaedic Disease (DOD). In adult horses it causes lameness and bone fractures. So little calcium and phosphorus in the diet that the bone fails to mineralise correctly is known as rickets in growing horses and osteomalacia in adult horses. In severe cases the bone becomes demineralised and fibrous tissue is deposited in its place, leading to enlargement of the facial bones called 'big head'. Horses working hard in hot conditions may lose large amounts of calcium in sweat leading to post-exertional hypocalcaemia; horses show muscle spasms, incoordination and synchronous diaphragmatic flutter.

Horses require a daily intake of 5g Ca and 2g P/100 kg body weight to balance daily losses and the efficiency of absorption from the gut. This approximates to 2.5g Ca/kg diet and 1g P/kg diet. The availability of calcium in feeds lies between 45–70 per cent and the amount of phosphorus will affect absorption from the gut. Thus the mature adult horse will require about 23g Ca and 18g P in the diet, met by 64g of limestone or 60g dicalcium phosphate. Although bonemeal is a good source of both calcium and phosphorus it is not recommended for feeding to horses in the light of the BSE problems.

Phosphorus is absorbed efficiently from both the small and large gut; calcium is mainly absorbed from the small intestine. This is a possible reason for the fact that excess phosphorus depresses calcium absorption: the phosphorus does not 'allow' the calcium to be picked up in the small intestine, so that it passes into the large gut, where it cannot be absorbed.

Limestone is calcium carbonate and only provides calcium, while dicalcium phosphate provides both.

**Table 2.2**   Minimum daily requirements for calcium and phosphorus.

| Age | Body weight (kg) | Calcium (g) | Phosphorus (g) | Limestone (g/day) | Dicalcium phosphate (g/day) |
|---|---|---|---|---|---|
| 3 months | 100 | 37 | 31 | 104 | 148 |
| 6 months | 200 | 33 | 27 | 92 | 108 |
| 12 months | 300 | 31 | 25 | 87 | 92 |
| 18 months | 375 | 28 | 23 | 78 | 72 |
| Mature | 450 | 23 | 18 | 64 | 60 |
| Lactating | 500 | 33 | 23 | 92 | 108 |

## Magnesium (Mg)

Magnesium is associated with calcium and phosphorus metabolism and is a co-factor and activator for enzymes of the metabolic pathways of proteins, fats and carbohydrate. It is also needed for normal cell metabolism, and nerve and muscle function.

A deficiency is associated with mental apprehensiveness, excitement and muscular spasm and twitching. Good natural sources of magnesium include alfalfa, clover, bran and linseed. It can be added to diet as calcined magnesite, magnesium carbonate or magnesium sulphate.

## Potassium (K)

Potassium is important in body fluid regulation, acid-base balance, nerve and muscle function and carbohydrate metabolism. A deficiency is very rare because grass and conserved forages, e.g. hay, contain high levels of potassium. Losses during sweating or diarrhoea increase the need for potassium significantly. Horses in hard work tend to eat less hay, thus lowering dietary potassium along with increased losses in sweat; potassium should be replaced by adding a suitable electrolyte supplement to the diet.

### Sodium (Na)

Sodium, like potassium, is important in regulating the body fluid and the acid-base balance of the body. It is also involved in the transmission of nerve impulses and the absorption of sugars and amino acids from the gut. Deficiency of sodium results in body dehydration, poor growth and reduced utilisation of digested proteins and energy. Most natural feedstuffs fed to horses are low in sodium which means that the horse's diet should be supplemented with common salt (NaCl) by using a salt or mineral lick in the manger or adding salt to the feed. Diets containing 5–10 g common salt/kg will meet the normal sodium requirement. The working horse may lose 100 g salt/day through sweat, and this must be replaced to avoid dehydration.

### Chloride (Cl)

Chloride is closely associated with sodium and potassium in their role in body fluid regulation. Where the requirements for sodium are met it is unlikely that chloride will be deficient.

## The trace elements

### Copper (Cu)

Copper interacts with sulphur and molybdenum; deficiencies of copper in cattle have been associated with an excess of molybdenum in the soil. The horse appears to be better than cattle and sheep at withstanding copper deficiency but the signs of deficiency are anaemia, poor growth, hair depigmentation and weight loss. A lack of copper has also been implicated in some bone disorders. Copper is involved in the formation of bone, cartilage, elastin and hair pigment, and in the utilisation of iron during the production of haemoglobin and red blood cells.

The amount of copper in feedstuffs is directly related to the levels of copper in the soil on which the feed was grown, as well as to the feed type. High levels are found in seeds and seed by-products.

There is some evidence that what were formerly regarded as satisfactory blood copper levels are in fact too low, and that there is a relationship between low blood copper levels and poor performance in racehorses, which can be overcome by feeding a high copper feed supplement.

Ruminants store copper in the liver, making them prone to copper poisoning; however, very high levels of copper are necessary to increase copper levels in the livers of horses, making them more tolerant of copper in the diet. In order to allow for interaction with other minerals and to maximise iron retention, 15–20 mg/kg dry feed is needed by growing horses.

### Zinc (Zn)

Zinc is involved in normal cell metabolism and is an enzyme activator and antagonist. It is a co-factor in over 200 enzymes; as a result, deficiency has widespread physiological effects, such as skin lesions and reduced appetite and growth. The horse's dietary requirement is probably less than 50 mg/kg. High zinc levels interfere with copper utilisation and are associated with lameness and bone abnormalities, especially epiphysitis. Zinc is found in yeast, bran and cereal germ.

### Manganese (Mn)

Manganese is needed for the activation of the enzymes involved in cartilage formation. Uptake of manganese is impeded by a high calcium intake, which can result in a deficiency causing abnormal skeletal development and reproductive failure. Wheat bran contains good levels of manganese but the content in grass, and thus hay, varies widely.

### Iron (Fe)

Iron is essential for normal haemoglobin and red blood cell production; consequently a deficiency of iron causes anaemia. Most natural feeds, except milk, contain iron, so horses fed a normal diet are unlikely to be deficient unless they are heavily parasitised.

Fifty milligrams of iron per kilogram dry matter should be adequate for growing foals with 40 mg/kg meeting the maintenance requirements of adult horses. The use of iron supplements will not increase the horse's red blood cell count or haemoglobin concentration; indeed toxicity and harmful inter-reactions with other trace elements may occur.

## Iodine (I)

Iodine is involved in the synthesis of the hormone, thyroxine, that controls the rate of chemical reaction in the body. A deficiency or excess results in cell reaction rate abnormalities. Mares may have abnormal oestrous cycles, and will not conceive or will give birth to weak foals. There are trace levels of iodine in most feeds, especially of marine origin, e.g. seaweed. Diets supplemented with 0.1–0.2 mg I/kg should meet the requirements of horses.

## Selenium (Se)

Selenium is vital for the maintenance of normal muscle tissue and is closely related to vitamin E as a cell membrane stabiliser and protector. The requirement for both vitamin E and selenium is increased if the diet is high in cod liver oil, linseed or corn oil. A deficiency of selenium results in pale, weak muscle in foals and occasionally white muscle disease in adult horses. Low blood selenium levels have been associated with poor performance in racehorses. Excess selenium is toxic, causing mane and tail hair loss, hoof deformities, joint stiffness, lethargy, anaemia and weight loss. Horses require about 0.15 mg of available selenium per kilogram of feed; this requirement may not be met in horses grazing and eating feed grown on selenium-deficient soils.

Soils subject to high rainfall, waterlogging and a low soil pH tend to produce selenium deficient pasture, such as areas of the Welsh Hills, Shropshire, north Cornwall and the Scottish borders. Selenium deficiency also occurs on sands and gravels in, for example, Newmarket. Some areas of the USA and Eire may have toxic levels of selenium in the soil. Sources of selenium are linseed or commercial products available as specialised supplements.

## Chromium (Cr)

Chromium is essential for normal carbohydrate metabolism and is found in insulin-sensitive tissue where it reduces insulin resistance and stimulates glucose clearance. Chromium has recieved much interest in human nutrition, being used to help diabetics and obesity. It is thought that chromium supplementation may help energy metabolism in performance horses.

## Cobalt (Co)

Cobalt is vital for the synthesis of vitamin $B_{12}$ in the gut, and for the activation of enzyme reactions. A deficiency of cobalt leads to impaired vitamin $B_{12}$ production, and hence anaemia, loss of weight and reduced growth. A deficiency is rare because trace levels are present in most feeds.

**Table 2.3**   Minerals required by horses.

| Mineral | per kg of diet | per day for 16 hh 500 kg horse |
|---|---|---|
| Sodium (g) | 3.5 | 44 |
| Potassium (g) | 4.0 | 50 |
| Magnesium (g) | 0.9 | 11 |
| Sulphur (g) | 1.5 | 19 |
| Iron (mg) | 150 | 1900 |
| Zinc (mg) | 60 | 750 |
| Manganese (mg) | 50 | 625 |
| Copper (mg) | 20 | 250 |
| Iodine (mg) | 0.15 | 1.9 |
| Cobalt (mg) | 0.2 | 2.5 |
| Selenium (mg) | 0.2 | 2.5 |

# Vitamins

Vitamins are required in tiny amounts compared with other nutrients; nevertheless, a deficiency in the diet will result in disordered metabolism and eventually disease.

Some compounds function as vitamins only after undergoing a chemical change: these compounds are called provitamins or vitamin precursors, e.g. beta-carotene becomes vitamin A. There are at least 15 vitamins which are accepted as being essential to the horse; only those of major nutritional importance are mentioned here. Requirements vary from horse to horse and are entirely individual, which makes prescribing one vitamin supplement as being 'the best' very difficult.

Vitamins may be divided into two groups: fat-soluble and water-soluble. The fat-soluble vitamins can be stored in the horse's body, particularly the liver. Most of these (or their provitamins) are abundant in fresh green herbage. This means that the horse can take in more than it needs in the summer and store the vitamins for use in the winter. Stabled horses that have limited access to grass may not be able to store adequate amounts and may require supplementary cod liver oil, which is rich in vitamins A and D. Their coat condition will also benefit. The vitamin content of feeds varies according to the soil type, climatic conditions, harvesting and storage conditions. High quality leafy forage and sunshine give the horse many of the vitamins he requires, but deficiencies can occur if poor quality forage or high quantities of unsupplemented refined feeds are given. Additional vitamins may be necessary during drought conditions, if the horse is growing rapidly or is under stress.

The majority of water-soluble vitamins are synthesised by the microorganisms found in the horse's gut; this means that they do not need to be stored. Many of them are involved with the metabolism or utilisation of the fats, protein and carbohydrate that the horse eats; this means that the performance horse on a high energy diet may need higher levels of these vitamins. However as the horse gets fitter he eats less forage, he loses his grass-belly and the capacity of his hind gut shrinks and there are consequently fewer 'bugs' providing the vitamins. We may need to provide this horse with a suitable vitamin supplement.

## The water-soluble vitamins

### Vitamin B₁ (thiamine)

Thiamine was the first vitamin to be studied in detail. It was found that the disease beri-beri, seen in people eating polished rice, could be prevented if the rice bran was added back to the diet.

Thiamine is an essential part of many enzyme systems, particularly those that regulate the release of energy from stored carbohydrates and fat. Any shortfall of thiamine can be seen as a lack of energy, muscle weakness and cramp. A slight deficiency may lead to decreased feed consumption, with a resulting drop in condition, eventually leading to lack of coordination, weakness and diarrhoea.

Deficiency is rare unless the horse is consistently fed poor quality hay or eats bracken (*Pteridium aquilana*) which contains a vitamin B₁ antagonist. Bracken poisoning is reversed by removing bracken from the diet and giving large doses of vitamin B₁.

Thiamine is found in yeast, alfalfa, green leafy crops, peas, beans and cereal germ. It is also synthesised by bacteria in the horse's hind gut, but this production may not be adequate to meet the horse's requirement. Carbohydrate metabolism increases during exertion, so it is important that the performance horse has adequate levels of thiamine in the diet.

It is important to note that antibiotics can affect the synthesis of several B vitamins by upsetting the bacterial population of the hind gut.

## Vitamin B₂ (riboflavin or lactoflavin)

Initially riboflavin was also extracted from rice bran. It is a fundamental component of many enzymes involved in protein and carbohydrate metabolism but it cannot be synthesised by the horse. A deficiency of riboflavin leads to decreased energy production and protein utilisation, which means that growth and condition are adversely affected. Severe deficiency eventually results in periodic opthalmia (moon blindness), which leads to conjunctivitis in one or both eyes and profuse weeping of the eyes.

Good sources of riboflavin are green forage, milk and milk products. Good quality grass and hay should provide much higher levels than the estimated requirements.

## Vitamin B₃ (niacin)

Niacin is the active group of two important co-enzymes which catalyse the transfer of hydrogen in the metabolism of carbohydrates, fats and proteins. A lack of niacin leads to disorders of the skin, gut and nervous system. The first signs of deficiency are loss of appetite, reduced growth and diarrhoea. As the condition advances the skin may become scaly, the mouth ulcerated and the nervous system upset.

Niacin is widely found in feeds, in particular in lucerne, oil seeds and animal by-products. If a good quality diet is fed, a niacin deficiency is unlikely.

## Vitamin B₅ (pantothenic acid)

Pantothenic acid was first found in yeast and was shown to be an essential part of energy metabolism. It is also involved in the metabolism of fatty acids and in the formation of antibodies, which help combat disease. Deficiency of pantothenic acid causes weight loss, growth failure, dermatitis and skin disorders.

The synthesis of this vitamin in the gut should normally meet the horse's requirement and as peas, molasses, yeast, and cereal grains are all sources of pantothenic acid, deficiency is consequently rare.

## Vitamin B₆ (pyridoxine)

Pyridoxine is involved in a number of enzyme systems which are essential for protein and carbohydrate metabolism. It is also involved in central nervous system activity, blood haemoglobin production and disease prevention. This wide range of activity means that deficiency signs are non-specific and have not been reported in horses. Forages, grains and pulses all contain pyridoxine.

## Vitamin $B_{12}$ (cyanocobalamin)

For many years vitamin $B_{12}$ was known as 'the animal protein factor', as it is part of the enzyme system involved with protein metabolism. It contains cobalt and is needed for the production of red blood cells. A deficiency leads to loss of appetite, poor growth rates and anaemia (reduced red blood cell numbers). Mature horses are less susceptible to deficiency than youngsters.

Vitamin $B_{12}$ is synthesised exclusively by micro-organisms in the horse's gut; its presence in food is of microbial origin. Diets low in feeds of animal origin predispose the horse to deficiency as good sources are fish meals and meat and bone meals.

Cobalt is necessary in the diet at a minimum rate of 0.1 mg/kg diet for microbial synthesis of vitamin $B_{12}$. Supplementation may lead to a stimulation of appetite; loss of appetite may occur in horses on high grain diets due to a build up of blood proprionate and these horses may benefit from vitamin $B_{12}$ supplementation.

## Vitamin $B_{15}$ (pangamic acid)

Vitamin $B_{15}$ has been isolated from apricot pits but it is not recognised by the US Food and Drugs Administration as there is no exact chemical formula for it. Allegedly vitamin $B_{15}$ increases the supply of blood oxygen to the horse. The signs of vitamin $B_{15}$ deficiency are not known.

## Folic acid

Folic acid is intimately linked to vitamin $B_{12}$ and it is vital for red blood cell production. A deficiency is characterised by anaemia and poor growth. Folic acid deficiency may respond to vitamin $B_{12}$ supplementation.

Folic acid is widely found in horse feeds including good quality pasture, hay etc, cereals, and extracted oilseed meals. It is also synthesised in the horse's gut but as the requirement increases with exercise, performance horses may need a supplement of folic acid.

A daily supplement of 1 mg folic acid for foals and working horses is sufficient.

## Biotin

Biotin is one of the more recently discovered vitamins and until recently it was thought that horses could synthesise adequate amounts of biotin in the gut. It is a sulphur-containing vitamin which is involved in fat, protein and carbohydrate metabolism, although its complete role is not yet understood. It has been found that a lack of biotin causes skin changes, poor hoof horn and faulty keratinisation, which has led to biotin being given to horses with poor feet. As no specific requirement for biotin has been established, it is not possible to say whether or not horses that respond to biotin treatment had been on a biotin-deficient diet, but it seems that biotin may have a role to play in strengthening the hooves of horses with a history of foot weakness. The horse may need up to 20 mg of biotin daily for three years for maximum benefit.

Biotin is present in bran and barley but is unavailable to the horse. Maize, yeast, grass are available sources. The role of biotin is positively linked with the sulphur-containing amino acid, methionine.

## Choline

Choline is essential in building and maintaining cell structure and has important roles in fat metabolism and nerve transmission. Deficiency leads to slow growth and increased fat deposition in the liver. The requirement for choline is large but a deficiency is not usually seen because it is widely distributed in feedstuffs. It can also be made from the amino acid methionine; rations low in methionine may predispose the horse to choline deficiency. Green leafy forages, yeast and cereals are all good sources of choline.

## Vitamin C (ascorbic acid)

Sailors who had scurvy discovered that fresh fruits such as lemon or lime, which are high in vitamin C, prevented the disease. The role of the vitamin is normal collagen formation, maintenance and repair. Collagen is vital to the structure of skin and connective tissue. It is also involved in the transfer of iron from blood to body stores. As the sailors found, a deficiency leads to impaired collagen formation and thus delayed wound healing, oedema and weight loss.

The horse can synthesise its own vitamin C and it is generally assumed that this is adequate, although there is no clear proof. Good sources include green leafy forage.

## The fat-soluble vitamins

### Vitamin A (retinol)

In the early part of this century, the yellow pigment found in carrots, called carotene, was shown to be essential for life and health. It was then discovered that carotene is converted to vitamin A in the intestinal wall. Vitamin A is necessary for vision, the health of mucous membranes, growth, reproduction and resistance to disease. A deficiency leads to reduced sight and eye damage resulting in night blindness. Poor and uneven hoof growth, slow growth, reproductive failure and susceptibility to disease are other deficiency signs. Problems are most likely to occur if poor quality forage is consistently fed, or during drought conditions. Young horses will show a deficiency more quickly than adult horses.

Good sources of vitamin A include green, leafy forages and carrots. Grazing horses obtain vitamin A from carotenoids in herbage, principally beta-carotene. However, hay provides very little, if any, carotene. Horses kept on hay during the winter, with no access to pasture, may deplete their stores of vitamin A within two months of being stabled.

It is recommended that a 500 kg adult horse receives 15 000 iu of vitamin A per day; as most commercial feeds are supplemented at a rate of about 10 000 iu/kg, the majority of horses will be receiving much more than this.

Beta-carotene appears to have functions in addition to the formation of vitamin A, with evidence that it may stimulate fertility.

It is wasteful, expensive and potentially dangerous to overfeed excess vitamin A, leading to bone fragility and skin damage.

### Vitamin D (calciferol)

Vitamin D has two forms, $D_2$ (ergocalciferol) and $D_3$ (cholecalciferol); $D_3$ is the most effective form. Its main function is the absorption, uptake and

**Table 2.4**   Vitamin content of common feeds.

|  | Vitamin A (carotene) (mg/kg) | Vitamin E (tocopherol) (mg/kg) |
|---|---|---|
| Ryegrass | 260 | 40–100 |
| Lucerne | 180 | 37–110 |
| Leafy grass hay | 40 | 16–40 |
| Mature hay | 10–20 | 1–20 |
| Carrots | 890 | 1–5 |
| Maize | 2.5 | 4–18 |
| Barley | 0 | 2–14 |

transport of calcium and phosphorus. Deficiency or excess of vitamin D results in swollen joints, skeletal abnormalities, lameness. Excess also causes bone to be laid down in soft tissue. Horses that are rugged and housed, receiving little sunlight and eating a cereal-based diet are most at risk.

In the absence of vitamin D the efficiency of calcium absorption from the intestine and the mobilisation of calcium from the bone are depressed and blood calcium levels fall, eventually leading to rickets in young horses and osteomalacia in adult horses.

If the horse's commercial feed contains 1000 iu/kg the requirement for vitamin D should be met.

Vitamin D occurs as two provitamins which need the ultraviolet portion of sunlight acting on the skin to be converted to the vitamin. These precursors are found in most forages. The vitamin rarely occurs in plants but colostrum, the first milk, is a rich source for the foal.

## Vitamin K

Vitamin K is required for effective blood clotting. A deficiency means that the blood takes longer to clot, but a deficiency is rare as the vitamin is made by the bacteria of the gut. Dicumerol, a blood anti-coagulant, interferes with vitamin K function, leading to extended blood clotting time. Some body storage of vitamin K is possible and it is found in green leafy material, e.g. lucerne.

## Vitamin E (tocopherol)

Vitamin E is a group name for several closely related substances: alpha-tocopherol is the most common form, with the highest vitamin E activity. Vitamin E is required as a non-specific biological antioxidant: in other words it protects the cells from damage by oxidation. It also acts with selenium as a body tissue 'stabiliser', ensuring the stability of red blood cells and maintaining the integrity of the vascular system. A shortage of vitamin E leads to a wide variety of problems, including pale areas of skeletal and heart muscle, red blood cell fragility and infertility.

Vitamin E is found in alfalfa, green fodder and cereal grains, although the type of tocopherol can vary, e.g. barley has mainly alpha-tocopherol but maize also has gamma-tocopherol. Typical rations for horses should contain 75–80 iu/kg; this should be higher for performance horses. Generally rations should be adequate in vitamin E, but if high levels of fat are included extra vitamin E should be fed; a further 5 mg/kg vitamin E

**Table 2.5**  Vitamin supplementation required by horses.

|  | Total requirement | Supplement should provide |
|---|---|---|
| Vitamin A (iu/kg) | 12 000 | 12 000 |
| Vitamin D$_3$ (iu/kg) | 1 200 | 1 200 |
| Vitamin E (mg/kg) | up to 200 | 100 |
| Vitamin K (mg/kg) | (unknown) | 1 (max) |
| Vitamin B$_1$ (thiamine) mg/kg | 15 | 2 |
| Vitamin B$_2$ (riboflavin) mg/kg | 15 | 3 |
| Vitamin B$_3$ (niacin) mg/kg | 25 | 20 |
| Pantothenic acid mg/kg | 15 | 10 |
| Folic acid mg/kg | 10 | 1 |
| Choline mg/kg | 200 | 100 |
| Pyridoxine mg/kg | 10 | 2 |
| Vitamin B$_{12}$ mcg/kg | 250 | 20 |
| Biotin mcg/kg | 200 | 100 |
| Vitamin C mg/kg | 250 | 100 |

should be added for each 1 per cent fat above 3 per cent in the ration. Stress, low selenium in feed and poor quality feed will increase the vitamin E requirement of the horse.

# Water

Water serves two basic functions for all animals:

- as a major component in body metabolism
- as an important factor in body temperature control.

Water is essential for life:

- all the biochemical reactions that take place in the body need water
- water acts as a solvent
- water helps transport semi-solid digesta through the gut
- it transports solutes in blood, tissue fluids, cells and excretions
- it allows excretion through urine and sweat
- it dilutes cell contents and body fluids so that relatively free movement of chemicals can occur; it acts as a transport medium for absorbed substances.

## Water absorption

Water is absorbed from most sections of the digestive tract. Following a meal water will flow into the gut to dilute the digesta and maintain the optimum consistency of the digesta throughout the gut. If water is drunk without any food being eaten, the water is absorbed more rapidly and completely. Other factors will affect absorption; for example poly-saccharides, such as pectin, tend to form gels in the gut. These hold water and reduce water absorption and are known as laxatives. Any factor resulting in diarrhoea will result in reduced water absorption.

The amount of water provided by green forage can be very substantial, the resting horse may not need to drink any water if the grass moisture content is over 70 per cent.

**Table 2.6**  Expected water consumption of adult animals in a temperate climate.

| Animal | Litres/day |
| --- | --- |
| Beef cattle | 22–66 |
| Dairy cattle | 38–110 |
| Sheep | 4–15 |
| Horses | 30–45 |
| Pig | 11–19 |

## Regulation of drinking

The regulation of drinking is a highly complex physiological process, induced as a result of dehydration of body tissues. However, drinking may also occur when there is no need to rehydrate tissues. When an animal is thirsty salivary flow is usually reduced, and dryness of the mouth may stimulate drinking. Most animals drink during or soon after eating and frequency of drinking and the amount drunk increase in hot weather.

## Water requirements

Water requirements are difficult to define because numerous dietary and environmental factors affect water absorption and excretion. The horse's water requirements will vary depending on:

- ambient temperature
- high humidity
- sweating
- physiological state, e.g. lactation
- water content of feed

Diets that are dry or high in salt will increase the horse's thirst. Adult horses are better at conserving body water than foals, so foals dehydrate more quickly than adults. Tropical breeds are more adept at minimising water loss than horses designed to live in temperate climates. A rise from 15°C to 20°C in temperature will increase water loss by 20 per cent and so increase an adult horse's water requirement by about 5 litres.

An adult horse needs about 5 litres of water per 100 kg of bodyweight for maintenance – this is about 25 litres (5 gallons) for a 16 hh horse. Horses at maintenance require a minimum of 2 litres of water per kg of dry food; young growing horses need 3 litres per kg of dry food. The lactating mare may be secreting 12–15 kg of water daily in her milk and needs 4 litres of water per kg of dry food. Strenuous effort in hot conditions can increase this requirement up to 12–15 litres per 100 kg bodyweight – 60–75 litres (12–15 gallons) for the 16 hh horse. If this requirement is not met fatal dehydration may result.

In the adult horse 70 per cent of water is lost in the faeces and urine, the rest being lost through the lungs and skin. Foals are not as good at concentrating their urine and faeces as adult horses, and dehydrate rapidly and may die when suffering from diarrhoea.

A natural source of water to horses is fresh grass. Rapidly growing spring grass may contain 80 per cent water, and if the weather is not too warm this may supply all the horse's water needs. Under most circumstances the horse should have free access to fresh, clean water at all times. However after hard, fast work during which the horse has been denied water, care should be taken to cool the horse before allowing it substantial amounts of water. Excessive consumption of cold water by hot horses can cause colic or laminitis.

## Sources of water

### The horse at grass

Rivers and streams can be a good way of watering horses at grass, provided that the river is running water with a gravel bottom and a good approach. Shallow water and a sandy bottom may result in small quantities of sand being ingested, collecting in the stomach and eventually causing sand colic.

Ponds tend to be stagnant and are rarely suitable; they are usually best fenced-off and alternative watering arrangements made.

Filled from a piped water supply, field troughs provide the best method of watering horses at grass. Troughs should be from 1 to 2 m (3 to

6 feet) in length and about 45 cm (18 inches) deep. There must be an outlet at the bottom so that they can be emptied and scrubbed out regularly. The trough should be on well-drained land, clear of trees so that the ground around the trough does not get poached and the water does not fill up with leaves. During the winter troughs should be checked twice a day and the ice broken if necessary. They must be free from sharp edges or projections, such as a tap, which might injure a horse. If the trough is tap-filled, the tap should be at ground level and the pipe from the tap to the trough fitted close to the side and edge of the trough. The best method is to have a self-filling ballcock arrangement in a closed compartment at one end of the trough. Ideally the trough should be sited along a fence or recessed into it, rather than at right angles to it or in front of it. If not in the fence line the trough should be three to four horse's lengths into the field so that there is free access all round and horses cannot be trapped.

In the absence of satisfactory chemical analysis of water supplies, mains water is most reliable. Deep wells and bore holes can provide equally good water, as long as the analysis shows them to be satisfactory throughout the year and as long as the supply is constant even in the driest summer. In industrial areas rivers, streams and ditches can be risky water sources because of pollution with sewage and industrial wastes, and in arable areas there may be seepage of nitrates and nitrites from highly fertilised arable crops after heavy rainfall. Rivers in hot summers and ditches in coastal areas can be brackish and contain salt. This water puts a burden on the kidneys; it does not allow the water requirement to be met and may cause diarrhoea.

Water should have a low concentration of dissolved constituents, but in the chalk downlands of the UK water may have high levels of calcium, supplying up to 20 per cent of the horse's daily calcium requirement. This may help prevent growth problems where the diet has been poorly designed and is low in calcium.

### The stabled horse

Stabled horses are usually offered water in a bucket or an automatic drinker; both of these have advantages and disadvantages.

Buckets can be placed on the floor, in the manger, hung in brackets or suspended from a hook or ring at breast height. They should be placed in a corner away from the manger, hay-rack and door, but should still be visible from the door for checking. Providing water in buckets is time-consuming and heavy work; they must be emptied, swilled out and refilled at least twice a day, and topped up three or four times. Horses frequently knock buckets over and may damage themselves by getting a leg caught between the bucket and the metal handle. The main advantage is that you can monitor how much the horse is drinking – a change in a horse's drinking habits may be the first sign of illness.

Automatic drinkers are expensive to install, but they are an asset in a large yard, saving time and effort. They should be fairly deep so that the horse can take a full drink and must be cleaned out regularly, sited away from the manger and hay-rack and well-insulated to stop the pipes freezing in winter. Some horses are reluctant to drink from them and water intake cannot be monitored.

**Table 2.7**   Minimum daily water requirements of mares.

| Weight (kg) | Last 90 days of pregnancy (gallons/day) | First three months of lactation (gallons/day) |
|---|---|---|
| 200 | 3 | 6 |
| 400 | 5 | 9 |
| 500 | 6 | 11 |

**Table 2.8**   Characteristics of a good water source.

| | mg/litre |
|---|---|
| ammonia (albuinoid) | less than 1.0 |
| permanganate value (taken after 15 mins) | less than 2.0 |
| Nitrite, N | less than 1.5 |
| Nitrate, N | less than 1.0 |
| Calcium | 50–170 |
| Lead | less than 0.05 |
| pH | 8.8–7.8 |

## The 'Rules of Watering'

(1)   A constant supply of fresh clean water should always be available.
(2)   If this is not possible, water at least three times a day in winter and six times a day in summer. In this situation always water before feeding.
(3)   Water a hot or tired horse with water which has had the chill taken off it.
(4)   If a bucket of water is left constantly with the horse, change it and swill out the bucket at least twice a day, and top it up as necessary throughout the day. Standing water becomes unpalatable.

(5) Horses that have been deprived of water should be given small quantities frequently until their thirst is quenched. They must not be allowed to gorge themselves on water.

(6) During continuous work water the horse as often as possible, at least every two hours. Hunters should be allowed to drink on the way home.

(7) If horses have a constant supply of fresh clean water there should be no need to deprive the horse of water before racing or fast work. However, the horse's water can be removed from the stable two hours before the race, if thought necessary.

# Chapter 3
# Feeds and Feed Values

Horses have traditionally received a diet of hay, oats and bran – the amount of concentrate fed depending on the amount and type of work done. Things are not quite as simple these days, with many different types of feeds and supplements available to the horse owner. In order to make a decision about what to feed, many things must be taken into consideration, for example:

- cost
- availability
- the horse's nutrient requirements
- quality
- the nutrient content of the feed.

Horse feeds fall into two main categories:

- roughage
- concentrates.

## Roughage

The digestive system of the horse is designed to suit a grazing life-style: eating frequent small meals of highly fibrous grass and other forages. This means that the roughage part of the horse's diet is the most natural element – yet it is often the most neglected and poorest quality part of the stabled horse's daily food.

For many years grass and other forages have been conserved for winter use as hay; now there are alternative forages such as silage and haylage available for feeding horses.

## Hay

Grass hay falls into two types, meadow hay and seed hay.

### Meadow hay

This is made from well established permanent pasture that has probably been grazed at some point, and usually contains a mixture of grasses, for example fescues (*Festuca*), ryegrasses (*Lolium*), meadow grasses (*Poa*), foxtails (*Alopecurus*), timothy (*Phelum pratense*) and cocksfoot (*Dactylis glomerata*). The legume white clover (*Trifolium*) is usually also present. Meadow hay is generally softer and potentially lower in protein than seed hay.

### Seed hay

Seed hay is made from ryegrass based leys, the primary function of which is to be cut for hay-making. There is usually a majority of ryegrasses (Italian and perennial) along with a little clover. If the ley is designed to be used for grazing after the hay has been cut, a little timothy may be added to the seed mixture to extend the growing season. Seed hay is generally coarser in texture and potentially higher in protein than meadow hay.

The quality of the hay depends on how the hay is made; as long as the hay is composed of safe, nutritious plants, the stage of maturity at the time of cutting and the weather conditions during hay-making are much more important to the final outcome than the types of grass present. Poorly-made seed hay will be less nutritious than well made meadow hay.

### Factors affecting hay quality:

- variety of grass
- time of cutting
- the drying process
- storage.

### Variety of grass

The varieties of grasses present in the sward will affect the quality of the hay; some grasses are naturally more productive and nutritious than others. The most nutritious part of a forage is the leaf, containing about 60 per cent of the energy and 75 per cent of the protein. As the grass ages it becomes more lignified and stemmy, and consequently less nutritious. After seeding the fibre in the grass increases and the protein levels drop. In seed hay the varieties of grass will come to maturity at the same time and it is therefore easier to cut the crop before the grass seeds.

The best time to cut hay is just at the onset of flowering; this gives the optimum quantity with a reasonably high protein level of 9–10 per cent of the dry matter. If possible the grass should be cut when the sun is on it as there will be more sugars in the leaves. Meadow hay contains a variety of grasses which will all head at different times; at cutting, some grasses will have just flowered while others will have seeded and gone past their best. This means that the quality of meadow hay can be very variable.

If a pasture is grazed early in the year and then rested before taking a hay crop, this will encourage early flowering and may lead to a more stemmy hay with lower protein content.

### Time of cutting

Many hay producers are tempted to leave hay crops longer before cutting in order to get a better yield of hay. Unfortunately the grass will have lost much of its nutritional value; the crude protein may drop to 3.5–6 per cent with high fibre levels.

### The drying process

The drying process can be equally influential on hay quality. Hay which is dried in the field needs to be turned to ensure that it is thoroughly dry. Brittle dry leaves can be broken and lost during this process, reducing the feed value of the hay. The same is true for seeds that have shrunk during the drying process: these may fall out leaving only the empty flower heads and stalks. Rain falling on cut grass will wash nutrients out of the hay and prolong the hay-making process.

These problems can be overcome by barn-drying hay; the cut grass is artifically dried inside before baling. The resulting hay tends to be higher in nutrients and the cost of drying can be partially offset against the saving in concentrate feed that should be possible. Barn-drying reduces the risk of hay being spoilt in the field by rain or by baling with too high a moisture content.

### Storage

The moisture content of hay needs to be reduced to 5–15 per cent for field-dried hay and 30–40 per cent for barn-dried hay. If the moisture content is higher than this and the hay is baled and stacked then it will undergo considerable heating as the grass continues its metabolic processes. This heating can be extreme enough to cause spontaneous combustion of the stack of hay. Hay that has heated in the stack is said to be 'mow-burnt'; it is a brownish colour with a characteristic malty smell due to mould formation in the hay. While horses sometimes find this hay quite palatable, it is of low nutritional value as the moulds have used up the sugar in the grass.

Hay baled with a moisture content of more than 15 per cent stands a good chance of heating. Once it is baled, the first 10–20 days see an increase in the acidity of the hay and rapid mould growth. The resulting heat is rarely enough to set the stack on fire but it will actually dry the hay. Gradually the temperature of the hay will drop, by which time mould formation is complete. If the weather is hot and dry, hay containing 15 per cent moisture may take until February to heat.

Mouldy hay should never be fed to horses; as long ago as 1788 a veterinary surgeon called J.A. Clarke recognised the involvement of mow-burnt hay in cases of broken wind. The climate in this country is not ideal for hay-making and 60–80 per cent of British hay is baled too damp and becomes significantly contaminated by mould; compared to only five per cent in Kentucky, USA.

An additional complication associated with mould is the presence of forage mites; these feed on the fungal spores and cause respiratory problems in their own right.

*What to look for in good hay*

- greenish-yellow but not brown
- sweet smell, not musty or malty
- free from dust when shaken
- plenty of leaf and cut before seeding.

When checking a bale, take a section or good handful from the centre of the bale; examine it for leaf and flower and test its 'nose' by smelling it. Do not attempt to 'nose' a mouldy sample. It is often easy to see the dust that is released when the sample is taken from the bale but it can be startling to shake out a section of hay onto a white sheet – even what you thought was good hay can be loaded with spores and dust. If you are in doubt about the quality of the hay get a vet or nutritionist to check the hay for fungal spores and the nutrient content; the spores can be seen clearly under a microscope (Figs. 3.1, 3.2, 3.3).

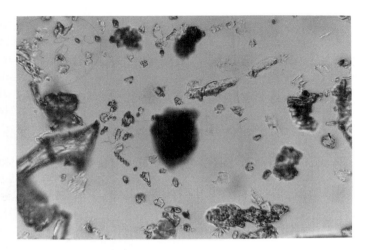

**Fig. 3.1**   Clean hay viewed through a microscope.

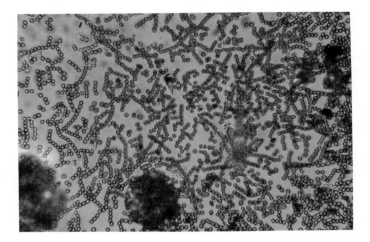

**Fig. 3.2**   Dirty hay viewed through a microscope.

## The feeding value of grass hay

Hay that is properly produced and correctly stored is a valuable part of the horse's diet. It can supply all the nutritional requirements of a horse on a maintenance ration. Poor quality hay not only necessitates the feeding of additional concentrates, but in some cases can be detrimental to the horse's health, resulting in long term or permanent problems.

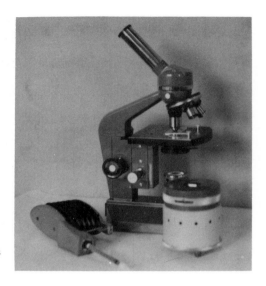

**Fig. 3.3** Fungal spore analysis equipment.

The values in Table 3.1 are only guidelines and a nutrient analysis will allow you to determine your hay quality and balance the ration accordingly.

Ideally new hay should be left about 12 weeks before feeding it; if this is not possible try to mix old and new and watch the bales carefully for signs of heating.

## Legume hays

Legumes are plants that, with the help of bacteria, are able to 'fix' nitrogen from the soil. Nitrogen is an essential part of protein, consequently

**Table 3.1**   Composition of hay and other high fibre feeds.

| Feed | Crude protein (%) | Crude fibre (%) | Digestible energy (MJ DE/kg) | Dry matter (%) | pH |
|---|---|---|---|---|---|
| Hay | 4.5–10 | 30–40 | 7–10 | 80 | |
| Silage | 10 | 30 | 10 | 25 | |
| Haylage | 8–14 | 30–38 | 9–11.5 | 55–65 | 5.3–5.8 |
| Straw | 3 | 40 | 6 | 88 | |
| Sugar beet pulp | 7 | 34 | 10.5 | Fed soaked | |
| Alfalfa chaff | 15–16 | 32 | 9–10 | 80 | |
| Alfalfa/straw chaff | 10.5 | 38 | 7 | 80 | |
| High fibre cubes | 9 | 20 | 8.5 | 85 | |
| Grassmeal | 16 | 36 | 9–10 | 85 | |

legumes have higher protein levels than most grasses. Legumes used for hay include clover and sainfoin, but more commonly alfalfa or lucerne. Moisture loss from the thick stems of lucerne is slow, the leaf dries more quickly and tends to shatter more readily than grass leaves, so care is needed when the hay is turned in the field, otherwise nutrients are lost. At the same stage of maturity legume hays contain more digestible energy, protein, calcium, beta-carotene and some B vitamins than does grass hay.

Lucerne is grown in East Anglia but little field dried lucerne hay is made in the UK; it is more successfully used for chaff and haylage.

The poor hay-producing climate of the UK has led to the development of different ways of conserving forage for winter use, including silage and haylage.

## Silage

Silage, if well-made, is virtually dust and fungal spore-free; however feeding silage is often not a practical proposition for horse owners for two reasons:

- Silage is made in silos, clamps or big bales; these methods pose considerable logistical problems – how do you get the silage to the horse?
- The packaging and storage of silage are vital; if done incorrectly potentially lethal micro-organisms can develop.

Ensiling a crop involves 'pickling' it in its own juice. The crop, usually grass or maize in the UK, is cut and left to partially dry or 'wilt' in the field, until the moisture content has dropped to 60–75 per cent. Grass is usually cut at or just after heading: in other words, the seed heads have appeared but the grass has not flowered. As many as four cuts may be taken from one field in one growing season if the grass is intensively grown; individual cuts are smaller but the total tonnage is greater.

The crop is then put into a silo, clamp or bag. Clamp silage is gathered from the field by a forage harvester that chops the grass so that when it is consolidated into a clamp, as much air as possible can be excluded. The clamp is covered and kept air-tight. The soluble sugars in the grass undergo fermentation, resulting in the production of acetic acid (vinegar) and an increase in acidity or lower pH. The acidity prevents the growth of harmful bacteria and fungal spores and preserves the grass. The dry matter content of the grass needs to be at least 25 per cent for this fermentation to drop the pH sufficiently; if the dry matter is only 15 per cent the pH will only fall to about 4.5, bacteria will grow and the silage will undergo a secondary fermentation resulting in a poor quality product that is not palatable to horses. Molasses and other additives are sometimes added to clamp silage to ensure that the correct fermentation takes place.

Big bale silage has a higher dry matter, often being wilted in the field to 40 per cent dry matter. It is then tightly baled and wrapped in plastic, or put in a tough plastic bag. A mild fermentation takes place resulting in a pH of 5–6. Additives are not used and it is the airtight environment and low water activity that preserves the grass and prevents bacterial proliferation.

If silage is readily available remember the following points:

- The silage should have been made to meet the nutrient demands of horses; silage made for beef and dairy cows tends to be too rich for horses.
- The acidity of the silage must be carefully monitored to check that a stable fermentation has taken place; the pH should be between 5 and 6 in big bale silage and 4–4.5 in clamp silage.
- The grass from which the silage has been made should be free of weeds, not cut too close to the ground and there should be no mole hills in the field.
- There must not be any mould.
- The dry matter should be a minimum of 25 per cent.
- The silage should have an attractive vinegary smell and must not smell of ammonia.

If these criteria are met then good quality silage can be a useful hay substitute, but always remember that there have been several deaths in the UK among horses eating big bale silage. These deaths were associated with toxins and bacteria that had proliferated due to abnormal fermentation in the silage.

## Hay alternatives

The British climate is not ideally suited to making hay and as a result horse owners may be faced with a shortage of good quality hay. The horse is designed to live on a high fibre diet; any shortfall of hay must be compensated for by adding another high fibre feed, for example:

- silage
- haylage

- straw
- chaffs
- sugar beet pulp
- high fibre cubes
- succulents, e.g. carrots.

Most of the hay alternatives mentioned have a better nutrient value than the hay they are replacing or supplementing and should be fed carefully; it may be necessary to reduce or change the concentrate ration. If hay is replaced by a more concentrated energy source, such as haylage, the horse will eat its day's ration of food more quickly and may become bored. All new feeds, including hay alternative such as haylage, straw and silage, should be introduced gradually into the horse's ration to avoid digestive upset.

## *Haylage*

Haylage lies between silage and hay in its feeding value and digestibility. It is highly palatable and horses can take in large amounts of energy quite rapidly, so care should be taken not to overfeed. Haylage should be substituted for hay on a weight for weight basis; it contains a lot of water and is consequently heavy, so that the horse will be receiving equivalent amounts of energy and protein from a smaller volume ration. The downside of this is that the horse will be receiving less fibre and the haylage will be eaten more quickly than the equivalent hay ration.

Correct fermentation is vital to preserve the haylage and also affects its suitability for feeding to horses. The following guidelines should be used:

- The dry matter should be between 45 and 65 per cent, preferably 55–65 per cent; however, forage with a dry matter of only 45 per cent can be considered if all the other parameters are satisfactory.
- The pH (acidity) should lie between 4.5 and 5.8. Silage or haylage with a pH of less than 4.5 is often unpalatable and may cause scouring; it can also be fatal to donkeys. Above a pH of 6 the silage or haylage will not be acidic enough to prevent the potentially lethal micro-organisms developing.
- The ammonia nitrogen level should be less than 5 per cent.

Some haylage is also produced specifically for horses. Grass is cut and allowed to wilt until the moisture content is down to about 45 per cent and then baled in the same way as hay. The bales are then compressed to about half their size and sealed in tough, plastic bags. Fermentation takes place which preserves the grass. Different types of bagged haylage are produced, for example alfalfa and high fibre types are available. Special closely woven haynets can be used to feed haylage, in order to slow down the horse's rate of eating.

## Feeding hay and alternative forages

1 kg hay contains on average 88 per cent dry matter, 6 MJ digestible energy, 5 per cent crude protein.

1 kg haylage contains on average 55 per cent dry matter, 5.5 MJ digestible energy, 6 per cent crude protein.

Thus if haylage is substituted for hay on a weight for weight basis, regardless of the fact that haylage contains a lot of water and consequently weighs heavy, then the horse will be receiving equivalent amounts of energy and protein. This calculation was based on average quality hay.

## Straw

Good quality spring barley or wheat straw in small quantities can act as a useful source of fibre for horses with sound teeth, but it is deficient in most nutrients. Fungal spores tend to be concentrated on the leafy part of plants. Straw has little leaf and it is easier to get clean straw than it is hay, which makes straw useful to feed as bulk to accompany a haylage or silage based ration. It is also a good filler for fat ponies that do too well on hay. Care must be taken to provide correct levels of minerals and vitamins if straw is to be used in the diet.

## Hydroponic grass

Hydroponic grass is the result of germinating barley seeds in lighted trays in a controlled humid environment in a specially designed cabinet (Figs. 3.4 and 3.5). The 'grass' is harvested when about six days old, and fed as a succulent feed with a feeding value similar to that of spring grass in terms of energy and protein. The grass is dust-free and highly digestible with good levels of vitamin E, beta-carotene and biotin. About 75 per cent of the grass is water, resulting in a digestible energy of about 2.5 MJ/kg – half that of hay or haylage, despite its high digestibility. The initial cost of the equipment and the labour needed to produce the grass make

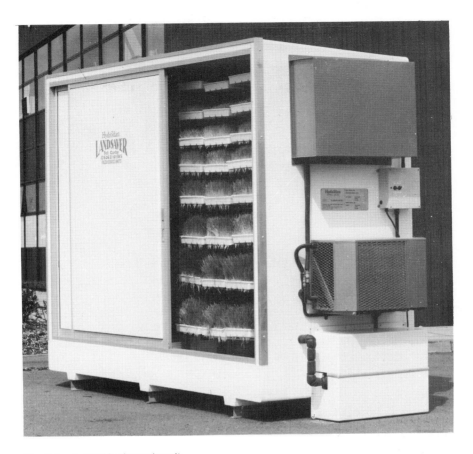

**Fig. 3.4**  A small hydroponic unit.

hydroponic grass expensive but the cost may be justified in some circumstances, e.g. stud farms with early foaling mares.

## Chaff

Traditionally a horse's concentrate feed was bulked up with chopped hay and/or straw to stop the horse bolting its feed and to encourage it to chew the feed more thoroughly. The modern equivalent takes the form of molassed chaff, and as the popularity of bran has waned, so the use of chaff has increased. Molassed chaff is particularly useful for horses and ponies on a very small concentrate ration. It prevents them from bolting the feed, provides fibre and soaks up any supplements the horse may be receiving. Fed with a horse and pony cube, it makes a simple ration that can be fed safely by the most inexperienced feeder.

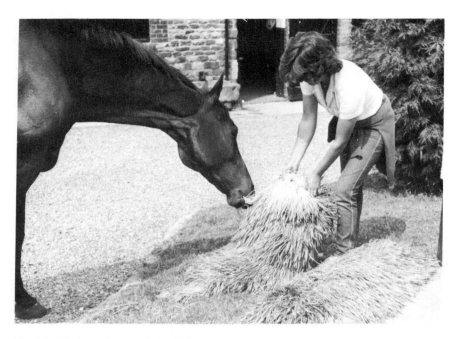

**Fig. 3.5**   Hydroponic grass being fed.

Most straw-based, molassed chaffs are designed to bulk out the hard feed and to slow down the horse's rate of eating. Hay and alfalfa or straw chaffs have been designed as partial or complete hay replacers, to be fed pound for pound for good quality hay. Alfalfa chaff is too high in energy and protein to be fed to most horses as a hay replacer, but is a useful 'top-up', especially for horses in hard work.

## Sugar beet pulp

Dried sugar beet pulp is a very under-estimated and under-utilised horse feed. Produced as either shreds or pellets, it is the dried remainder of the sugar beet once the sugar has been extracted. Once soaked, it makes a palatable and nutritious succulent for all types of horse and pony. Sugar beet pulp is economical and with a protein content of 7 per cent and an energy value similar to oats, it has the potential to be a significant part of the horse's ration. Instead it tends to be used as a feed-dampener, with horses rarely receiving more than a double handful in each feed. The high fibre content of beet pulp (34 per cent) means that it is a compromise between a forage and a concentrate. The sugar is digested easily in the small intestine giving 'instant energy', while the fibrous part is fermented in the hind gut, releasing nutrients more slowly. This makes it a good feed for endurance horses and hunters, which may go many hours between feeds. Very wet beet pulp is a useful way of encouraging the horse to rehydrate himself.

Sugar beet pulp should be soaked before feeding to prevent it swelling in the oesophagus, stomach or small intestine and causing problems. Shreds should be soaked overnight for use the following day, while pellets should ideally be soaked for 24 hours. Fresh beet pulp should be soaked every day as it can go off rapidly in warm weather. Shreds should be just covered with water so that a wet, firm feed results, not a sloppy mass. One kilogram of pellets should be soaked in 2 kg water.

Horses can be fed up to 1.8 kg (4 lb) dry weight of beet pulp per day; this amounts to about four scoops of wet sugar beet pulp and would replace 1.8 kg (4 lb) hay. Sugar beet pulp is also a useful source of calcium. Unmolassed sugar beet pulp is now available, reducing the soluble carbohydrate level of the diet.

### High fibre cubes

Most high fibre cubes are not designed to replace the entire hay ration; however, they can be used to supplement poor quality grazing and they can be added to the ration when hay is in short supply. High fibre cubes are also useful to maintain the condition of resting horses and ponies and those suddenly thrown out of work, when they can replace the concentrate ration.

### Succulents

Succulents such as carrots and swedes are useful for adding variety to the diet and to help alleviate the boredom factor. It is not recommended that more than 2 kg (4 lb) per day is fed. Potatoes should be avoided.

## Concentrates

### Energy feeds

Traditionally cereals have been the principal source of energy for horses in hard work. Cereal grains contain 12–16 MJ DE/kg of dry matter compared to about 8.5 MJ/kg in average grass hay; in other words 1 kg of cereals can replace up to 2 kg of hay in the ration – hence the name concentrate. As we demand a higher energy output from the horse we have to feed him more concentrated energy sources in order to keep the ration within his appetite; this also reduces his natural grass belly to give a trim athletic outline.

A cereal grain can be divided into three main parts: the husk (aleurone), the endosperm and the embryo (Fig. 3.6). The endosperm has a rich store of starch, used by the plant during its early rapid growth. The husk and embryo contain the majority of the protein content of the grain. Cereal proteins are not as nutritionally valuable as animal protein and oil-seed protein, because they are relatively deficient in the essential amino acids lysine and methionine. The quality of the protein is higher in oats than in barley and maize due to a slightly higher lysine content. Cereals contain about 1.5–5 per cent oil: oats are richer in oil than maize, which is, in turn, richer than barley. All cereal grains are very low in calcium, containing less than 1.5 g/kg, but they contain three to five times as much phosphorus. The phosphorus is principally in the form of phytate salts which reduce the availability of calcium and zinc, further increasing the horse's need for a calcium supplement.

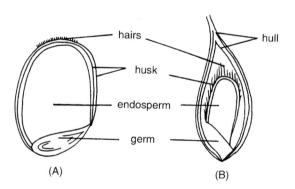

**Fig. 3.6**   Section through grain: (A) wheat and (B) oat.

## Oats

Oats are the traditional grain for horse feeding and can make up all of the concentrate ration. They have a relatively high fibre content and low energy content, which make them more difficult to overfeed. More oats can be fed before the horse suffers digestive problems such as laminitis. However they are known as being 'heating' and many horse owners are reluctant to feed them. The fibre is due to the outer hull or husk, which maize and wheat lose during harvesting. This makes oats relatively light and bulky. Oats can be fed rolled or crimped; however horses over 12 months old with sound teeth should be able to chew and digest whole oats effectively. Once rolled, oats begin to lose their nutritional value and should be fed as soon as possible. Try to avoid buying from a feed merchant who may have had rolled oats in stock for a long time.

Naked oats are a modern development of this traditional feed; the hull separates from the kernel during harvesting to leave a clean grain. Naked oats are more dense and have higher energy and protein levels than conventional oats. Fewer oats need to be fed to supply the same levels of energy in the diet and there is no need to crimp or roll naked oats. Naked oats are intended as a feed for performance horses; they can contain up to 27 per cent more energy than conventional oats. Great care must be taken when feeding them – they must be fed in smaller quantities and the forage level of the diet must be kept up.

**Table 3.2**  Nutrient values of commonly fed concentrate feeds.

| | Crude Protein (%) | DCP* (%) | Oil (%) | MAD† Fibre (%) | Ca (g/kg) | P (g/kg) | Lysine (g/kg) | DE (MJ/kg) |
|---|---|---|---|---|---|---|---|---|
| Oats | 9.6 | 7–8 | 4.5 | 17 | 0.7 | 3.0 | 3.2 | 11–12 |
| Naked oats | 13.5 | – | 9.7 | 3.2 | 0.2 | 0.4 | 5 | 16 |
| Barley | 9.5 | 7–8 | 1.8 | 7 | 0.6 | 3.3 | 3.1 | 13 |
| Maize | 8.5 | 7–8 | 3.8 | 3 | 0.2 | 3.0 | 2.6 | 14 |
| Linseed Extracted | 22 | 17 | 32 | 7.6 | 2.4 | 5.2 | 7.7 | 18.5 |
| Soyabean meal | 44 | 39 | 1.0 | 10 | 2.4 | 6.3 | 26 | 13.3 |
| Peas | 23 | 19 | 5 | 8.2 | 0.7 | 4.0 | 15.8 | 14 |
| Grassmeal | 16 | 11 | 3.2 | 36 | 6.0 | 2.3 | 8 | 9.6 |
| Alfalfa meal | 17 | 12 | 3 | 40 | 15.0 | 2.0 | 8.2 | 9 |
| Wheatbran | 15.5 | 10–12 | 3 | 12 | 1.0 | 12 | 6 | 11 |
| Sugarbeet pulp | 7 | 5 | 1.0 | 34 | 10 | 11 | 2.8 | 10.5 |
| Vegetable oil | 9 | 0 | 100 | 0 | 0 | 0 | 0 | 35 |
| Molasses | 3 | 1–2 | 0 | 0 | 7.2 | 1.0 | 0 | 11 |

*DCP = Digestible Crude Protein
†MAD fibre = Modified Acid Detergent Fibre

## Barley

Barley has a higher starch content and a greater weight per unit volume than oats, and the hull is smaller and more tightly attached to the grain. This means that barley should be crimped to rupture the hull before feeding it to horses, so that the digestive juices can penetrate the grain.

Barley is often processed to gelatinise the starch by steaming, micronisation or extrusion; these processes will be discussed later.

Barley has a higher energy content than oats and the protein is of slightly lower quality, due to a low lysine level; both the oil and fibre content are low. As a result barley is easier to overfeed, a 'scoop' of barley being both heavier and more rich in energy than a 'scoop' of oats. This has led to barley being known as a 'fattening' feed. Horses can receive all of their grain ration as barley provided that it is introduced into the diet gradually and that care is taken not to overfeed the horse.

Some horses may have a reaction against barley, resulting in filled legs or lumpy swellings. Take barley out of the ration and substitute another cereal or compound. These horses may not react to cooked or treated forms of barley.

*Maize*

Maize is a high energy, low protein, low fibre cereal and has a reputation for being 'heating'. In the UK it is generally fed steamed and rolled but it can be fed as whole grains if the horse has sound teeth. Maize can supply a large proportion of the energy in the horse's ration, provided that it is balanced by a quality roughage with a good protein level or by a high protein concentrate. Its price tends to mean that maize is only fed as a small proportion in the diet of horses that are not 'good doers' or need more condition.

*The 'heating' effect of grain*

Grain is often said to be 'heating', meaning that it results in a horse being overexcited and difficult to control. This heating effect stems from two sources:

*Overfeeding energy* – many 'hot' horses are simply getting too much energy for the job that they are doing and a reduction in the concentrate ration and an increase in the roughage will solve many problems. The behavioural problems are made worse by confining the horse to its stable 23 hours a day and then working the horse to increase its fitness – a veritable time bomb.

*Fermentation* – any grain passing through into the large intestine is rapidly fermented by the intestinal micro-organisms; there is an increase in the acidity of the caecum which may lead to discomfort, and the products of digestion pass very quickly into the bloodstream. There is a rise in blood levels of glucose and Volatile Fatty Acids which stimulates the metabolic rate thus 'heating' the horse both literally and mentally.

Processing cereals increases the amount of digestion in the small intestine, reduces caecal fermentation and keeps the horse's metabolism more stable.

## Protein feeds

As we have seen, the protein in hay can vary dramatically and the cereals do not generally have high protein levels; this means that horses with a high protein requirement such as broodmares and youngstock may require additional protein in the ration. Feeds high in protein include soyabean meal, linseed, peas, beans, yeast and high quality dried forage, particularly alfalfa.

### Soyabean meal

Oilseed meals like soyabean meal are much richer sources of protein than cereals, and the balance of amino acids is superior. Soyabean meal is considered to be the best quality vegetable protein fed to horses. Raw soya beans are poisonous but if reliably cooked, the meal can be used as the sole source of supplementary protein in the horse's ration. Soyabean meal contains 44–49 per cent protein; more expensive soya flakes are also available, containing 36–40 per cent crude protein. Feeding 1 kg of 40 per cent soyabean meal can raise the protein content of an oats-and-hay diet from 8 to 12 per cent, which would then provide adequate protein for a broodmare in mid-lactation.

### Linseed

Linseed should be cooked before feeding to horses, to destroy an enzyme that ultimately produces cyanide. Linseed has the ability to absorb large amounts of water, producing a thick gelatinous soup during cooking. This has a laxative effect and can sometimes overcome constipation without causing scouring. Linseed has a protein value of 20–22 per cent but it is generally fed in such small amounts that its contribution towards raising the protein of the ration is almost negligible. Its high oil content helps coat condition and it is a relatively good source of B vitamins.

Linseed cake is found in some coarse mixes but horses may not find it particularly palatable.

*Peas and beans*

Micronised field peas and field beans are frequently incorporated into coarse mixes and they can be bought as 'mixed flakes' along with maize. They contain 23–27 per cent protein and are a valuable source of the amino-acid lysine. The high protein and energy content of peas and beans makes them a useful ingredient in youngstock rations and they can be fed to performance horses if the quality of the forage is in doubt.

*Fishmeal*

Fishmeal is a high quality protein source, rich in minerals, trace elements and some water-soluble vitamins. It is expensive and is sometimes incorporated in foal creep feeds and mare's milk replacers.

Meat and unsterilised bone derivatives must not be fed to horses due to the risk of infection with Salmonella and Bovine Spongiform Encephalopathy (BSE).

*Milk pellets*

Milk pellets are based on dried skimmed milk, usually with added minerals and vitamins. Skimmed milk is virtually fat-free and consequently low in fat-soluble vitamins but the protein quality is high. Horses over three years old lose the ability to digest milk sugar, lactose, and will gain little energy from being fed dried skimmed milk. It is useful for foal creep feeds, but its use approaching weaning should be minimal, as the idea is to accustom the foal to feeds other than milk so that weaning is not so traumatic.

## Fillers and appetisers

This group of feeds may not contribute significantly to the nutrient requirements of the horse but they are still widely fed. Many horses are greedy and bolt their feed or are fussy and need to be tempted to eat; these feeds have a role to play in formulating practical and tasty rations.

### Wheatbran

The milling of wheat leads to a by-product called wheatfeed consisting of germ, bran, coarse middlings and fine middlings. Wheatgerm is generally too expensive to feed to horses but bran has long been fed as a source of roughage in the concentrate ration. Bran is actually lower in fibre than oats, containing 12 g/kg compared to 17 g/kg, and the fibre is not very digestible having a high level of indigestible lignin. The crude protein level of 14–16 per cent looks high but this too is not very digestible, with a digestible crude protein of 10–12 per cent. Bran is consequently expensive for the nutrients it provides, but a bran mash can make a palatable vehicle for the administration of oral medicines. Bran has the ability to hold much more than its own weight of water, which means that it has a laxative effect on the gut; this is useful if the horse suddenly has to be rested and there is a risk of azoturia.

Bran is deficient in calcium and very high in phosphorus, of which 90 per cent is in the form of phytate salts. These salts inhibit the uptake of calcium and phosphorus from the gut; not only is bran low in calcium it actually produces a calcium shortage which can cause bone problems, particularly in young, growing horses. A calcium supplement should always be fed if bran is included in the ration.

### Molasses

Molasses is the thick black liquid that remains after the sugar has been extracted from sugar beet or sugar cane. It contains minimal protein but a good energy level due to the sugar present. Its sweet taste is very attractive to horses, and molasses is used in many coarse mixes and cubes. It can be added to the concentrate ration at a rate of 0.5 kg per day to tempt the fussy feeder and to reduce the dustiness of the feed.

## Compound feeds – convenience feeds for horses

Compound feeds in the form of cubes and coarse mixes have been fed to horses for many years and make an appearance in most feed rooms these days. Compound feeds can be broadly divided into three groups:

- Complete cubes that are fed alone and replace all the hay and concentrates in the horse's ration. These cubes are high fibre and low energy, and can be used for native ponies to supplement grass or for horses that suffer from dust allergies to complement the semi-wilted bagged forage.
- Concentrate cubes that provide a balanced source of all the nutrients that a horse needs and are fed along with hay (or an alternative), water

and common salt. Different formulations are made for horses with different needs, so that cubes rich in nutrients and with high digestibility are made for foals, high energy cubes are given to horses in hard work and low energy cubes are given to those in light work.

- Balancer cubes or protein concentrates which are high protein cubes designed to be fed with cereals and forage and balance the deficiencies of the traditional part of the diet.

The advantages of feeding compounds:

- convenience
- standardised diets for specific purposes
- constant quality
- good shelf life
- dust-free
- palatable
- uniform weight and size, making the feeding routine more convenient
- economy of labour, transportation and storage
- no wastage.

The disadvantages:

- cannot tell good quality from poor quality ingredients
- the horse may find them boring to eat.

The first problem can be overcome by always using products from reputable compounders and seeking advice from their nutritionists. The label on the bag has by law to declare certain ingredients, and this can be a useful reference. The following information must be given:

- the percentage by weight of crude oil
- the percentage by weight of crude protein
- the percentage by weight of crude fibre
- the percentage by weight of total ash
- the amounts of added synthetic vitamins A, D and E (usually given as international units: iu per kg)
- the total selenium content if synthetic selenium has been added (mg/ kg)
- if an antioxidant has been added this must be stated
- some manufacturers now include digestible energy and digestible crude protein, which is very useful.

Remember that although straight feeds such as oats may look the same, you cannot see the protein and energy in them any more than you can in a cube. The bag that a cube comes out of states its feed value, a bag of oats does not have to do this.

Feed compounders range from large international feed manufacturers and merchants, producing rations for all types of livestock, with their own laboratories and nutritionists, through smaller specialist horse feed manufacturers to local feed mills. Cube manufacture is backed by extensive research facilities, the ability to bulk buy ingredients economically, and laboratory expertise which allows the analysis and balancing of ingredients of different quality. Oats can vary in their protein content by up to 8 per cent from one season to the next or one farm to the next. In order to meet the legally declared analysis, the manufacturer must analyse the oats and then add a suitable protein supplement to balance the compound.

Ingredients commonly used in cubes are ground cereal grains, oilseed meals, milling, brewing and distilling by-products, sugar beet pulp, dried grass and lucerne, fishmeal and minerals, trace elements and vitamin supplements. Coarse mixes contain cooked, flaked cereals and oilseeds and oil seed cake.

## The types of compound available

### Horse and pony cubes

Horse and pony cubes and mixes tend to be low energy, low protein and high fibre feeds; the basic nutrient specification of different brands of pony cube tends to be very similar. The cubes are designed to be 'non-heating', meaning that they will not oversupply the horse or pony in light work with energy, so that it is less likely to jump out of its skin. It is more difficult to make mistakes feeding horse and pony cubes; 1 kg may only contain 8 MJ DE, compared to a performance cube with up to 15 MJ DE per kg. One scoop of horse and pony nuts is equivalent to just over half a scoop of performance nuts on an energy basis.

### Performance feeds

Performance horse feeds are designed to meet the greater energy and protein requirements of the working horse. The analysis tends to vary much more than horse and pony cubes, so read the label carefully. The high protein versions are catering for the young racehorse that is still growing; the lower protein levels are better for adult performance horses. Some manufacturers have also taken on board the performance horse's need for certain minerals and vitamins and these are included at a higher level.

## Stud feeds

The lactating broodmare and the growing youngster do not need high energy levels, but have very high protein requirements to allow for rapid growth and milk production. This is where compounds come into their own; no single straight feed can supply enough protein without over-supplying the energy. Some manufacturers produce different rations for weanings and yearlings which reflect the changing nutrient requirements of youngstock.

## Feeding compounds

If we are honest few of us feed compounds as intended – we add oats or barley to them, believing that horses find them 'boring'; but we must be careful not to make our horses fussy – why should cubes, properly fed, be any more boring than grass? To combat this coarse mixes were produced: muesli for horses. We think that they look nice and are good enough to eat and we can see what is in them, enough to induce us to pay extra for them. However we continue to add grain to the mix, which unbalances the compound and defeats one of the reasons for feeding it – a convenient balanced ration in one bag. If you feel your horse needs more energy than the present cube is giving him, then buy a higher energy performance mix – there are plenty available.

## Balancer compounds

Many people appreciate the advantages of compounds, and yet have access to oats or prefer to feed them. The balancer is a protein con-centrate designed to be diluted with oats, and which contains higher levels of the appropriate minerals and vitamins. These balancers again come in different formulations to suit the differing requirements of stud stock, performance horses and horses in light work. Feeding a balancer allows you to overcome one of the main problems of feeding com-pounds, which is that no one feed can be correctly balanced for every horse all the time. Altering the ratio of balancer to oats as the horse's

**Table 3.3**  Typical nutrient values of compound feeds.

|  | Crude oil (%) | Crude fibre (%) | Crude protein (%) | Total lysine (%) | Digestible energy (MJ/kg) | Total ash (%) |
|---|---|---|---|---|---|---|
| Horse and pony cubes | 3 | 14–15 | 10 | 0.45 | 9 | 9–10 |
| Performance cubes | 3.5–4 | 8.5 | 12–13 | 0.55 | 12 | 8–10 |
| Stud cubes | 3 | 9–10 | 13–15 | 0.65 | 11 | 8–10 |
| Creep feed | 4–4.5 | 6.5–7.5 | 17–18 | 0.9 | 13 | 7–9 |
| Yearling cubes | 3–3.5 | 8.5 | 15–16 | 0.75 | 11 | 7–9 |
| Balancer | 3 | 10 | 17–19 |  |  | 15–18 |

condition changes lets the eye of the feeder and the art of feeding come into play.

Low energy balancers are also produced for horses and ponies that are prone to gain condition but still require minerals and vitamins to balance restricted intake of grass or hay. Balancers may also contain yeast preparations to enhance fibre digestion.

## High energy feeds

Several energy dense rations are produced for the performance horse market. These usually contain high levels of oil with additional vitamin E and are designed to be fed in small quantities to horses in hard work.

If you are in any doubt, ring the manufacturer and ask for help. Any reputable company will have a technical adviser who should be able to answer your questions.

# Feed processing

For years we have used boiled barley to put condition on lean horses; cooking it makes it more 'fattening'. Cooking methods have become more sophisticated and include steam flaking, micronisation and extrusion.

## Steam flaking

Barley and maize are often fed steamed and flaked. The grain is passed through heated rollers which cook and split the grain.

## Micronisation

A moving belt carries a thin, even layer of grain beneath a series of burners that emit infrared radiation; the grain is effectively 'microwaved' resulting in rapid internal heating and a rise in water pressure, which causes the starch in the grain to swell, break and gelatinise. The grain is then passed through rollers and cooled, emerging looking very similar to steam flaked grain. Steam flaked grain is usually slightly less brittle and dusty than micronised grain. Both processes are used to treat ingredients of coarse mixes, increasing digestibility and inactivating some toxic factors.

### Extrusion

Extrusion relies on high temperatures and the extreme buildup of steam to swell and cook a grain mixture. Grain or dry meal mixtures are impregnated with steam and water and then forced under very high pressure, in an oxygen-free environment, down a barrel by a screw feeder. Within 15–20 seconds the grain is heated from room temperature to over boiling point; it then passes out of the end of the barrel through a die-plate. The product is cut into shapes as it leaves the barrel, it expands and solidifies rapidly as the moisture in the product evaporates. The product is dried, cooled, sieved and bagged.

Extrusion and micronisation result in the unravelling of the complex starch molecule into a more easily digestible form. This effect is called gelatinisation and results in increased digestibility of the energy part of the grain without interfering with the digestibility of the protein. This means that there is less likely to be a high starch concentration in the large intestine, as more of it can be broken down and absorbed in the small intestine. The digestive upsets that can result from the rapid fermentation of starch in the caecum have been discussed and it is obviously a great advantage to avoid this potentially dangerous situation.

## Feed storage

Many of the nutrients in feeds deteriorate during storage and poor storage can speed up this effect. Not only will the feed be less nutritious but the horse will find it less palatable. All the fat-soluble vitamins A, D, E and K, occurring naturally in feed, will be oxidised together with poly-unsaturated fatty acids. The water-soluble B vitamins are fairly resistant during normal storage, although some will be lost if the feed is exposed to sunlight. Any storage advice on labels and bags should be followed.

Ideally a feedstore should have a low, uniform temperature and not be damp; there should be good ventilation, no direct sunlight and it should be free from birds and vermin. This means that when planning and building a feedstore it should be insulated, with no windows (but well lit and well ventilated), it should be easy to keep clean and free from leaks. Feed must be stacked on pallets so that it is raised off the ground and feedbins must be rodent-proof. Galvanised bins are preferable, as plastic can be chewed by rats. If you are using plastic bins make sure that you can check all sides of them easily and ensure that they are checked regularly. Probably the two most important criteria in siting a feedstore are that the area can be kept clean and rodent-free.

When sacks and bins are subjected to variations in environmental temperature they will 'sweat', i.e. there is moisture condensation, producing conditions ideal for mould growth. Insects such as mites and weevils accelerate the deterioration of feed and grain, generating heat and spreading fungal spores. Hygienic, low temperature dry storage areas are essential for successful long-term storage.

## Feed additives and prohibited substances

### Feed additives

Several drugs are used in the feed of farm animals to promote growth and to counteract disease. If using feed designed for animals other than horses, take care to check that they do not contain monensin or lincomysin, as these are poisonous to horses.

### Prohibited substances

Under the Rules of Racing and International Equestrian Federation (FEI) rules it is forbidden to give any stimulant, sedative or 'substance other than a normal nutrient' to a horse and detection of such a substance in the urine, blood, saliva or sweat of a horse will lead to disqualification. It is most unlikely that you will find any of the listed drugs in a horse's feed but occasionally contaminated feed ingredients have led to horses failing a dope test. Those substances causing the most concern are theobromine, caffeine and its metabolite, theophylline.

Caffeine is present in tea, coffee, cola nuts, cacao and mate leaves; if an ingredient destined for a horse feed is carried in the same hold on board ship that previously carried tea or coffee, the feedstuff will be significantly contaminated. The unwitting feeding of these substances through contaminated feed can result in a horse showing a positive dope test for up to 10 days.

Great care must be taken when feeding racehorses and competition horses, using only compound feeds that are guaranteed suitable for horses competing under FEI, British Showjumping Association (BSJA) or Jockey Club rules.

# Chapter 4
# Nutrient Requirements

## Estimating nutrient requirements

In the agricultural world animals are bred and fed to maximise production, be it eggs, meat or milk. Careful breeding programmes have led to animals that have a tremendous potential for production and extensive research has identified the feeding regime that will enable the animal to reach its potential.

In the wild, natural selection ensures survival of the fittest. The horse evolved to be athletic enough to evade predators, and to be an efficient converter of feed to allow it to survive the winter when forage was in short supply. During its years of domestication the horse has been bred for performance; how high the horse can jump or how fast it can run is more important than whether or not the horse is an efficient converter of feed. We can see this quite clearly when comparing the native breeds to the racing thoroughbred – there is no doubt which is the most efficient converter of feed.

The horse population varies widely, both between and within breeds, and as a result it is difficult to discuss the nutrient requirements of horses as a whole – all horses are individuals and should be treated as such. The problem is compounded by the fact that a horse is an expensive experimental animal, and comparatively little work has been done on its nutrient requirements.

A balanced ration provides energy, protein, fat, minerals, vitamins and water in sufficient quantities to keep the horse alive and allow it to do the work we demand. The nutrient demands of a horse will depend on many factors including:

- size
- condition
- work done
- appetite

- age
- reproductive status
- health
- environment
- management.

## Size

Obviously large horses need more food and eat more than small horses; in other words the horse's nutrient requirements and its appetite are closely related to its size. Size in this situation means bodyweight not height: a 14.2 hh cob weighs considerably more than a 14.2 hh show pony. This means that the first step in determining a horse's nutrient requirements and then designing a ration is to determine the horse's bodyweight. Bodyweight can be found out using:

- a weighbridge
- a tape measure and calculator
- a weightape
- a table of weights.

Few of us have access to an equine weighbridge so Milner and Hewitt (1969) devised an equation relating the horse's heart girth and the length from the point of shoulder to the point of the pelvis to the bodyweight (Fig. 4.1).

$$\text{Bodyweight (kg)} = \frac{\text{heart girth (cm)}^2 \times \text{length}}{8717}$$

or

$$\text{Bodyweight (lb)} = \frac{\text{heart girth (in)}^2 \times \text{length}}{241}$$

For example, a 16 hh middleweight horse which has a girth measurement of 165 cm (65 inches) and a length of 173 cm (73 inches).

$$\text{Bodyweight (kg)} = \frac{\text{heart girth (cm)}^2 \times \text{length}}{8717} = 540 \,\text{kg}$$

or

$$\text{Bodyweight (lb)} = \frac{\text{heart girth (in)}^2 \times \text{length}}{241} = 1280 \,\text{lb}$$

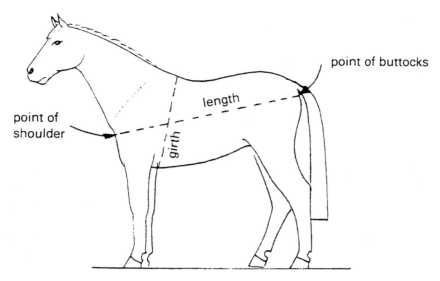

point of buttocks

point of shoulder

**Fig. 4.1**  Measurement of girth and length.

It is possible to buy a weigh tape which uses a measurement of the horse's heart girth to give an approximate bodyweight. Whilst not very accurate, this method is quick and easy to use and will help you record any changes in your horse's condition if measured on a regular basis.

## Food analysis

In order to make a successful ration it is important to know two things:

- the nutrient requirements of the horse
- the nutrient value of the feed given to the horse.

The nutrient values of feeds can be determined in the laboratory using a number of analytical procedures. Firstly the dry matter of the food is estimated, by removing all the water from a given weight of feed by drying it in an oven, and then reweighing it. Feeds with a high dry matter, like cereals, contain little moisture and each kilogram fed to the horse will contain more feed value. Feed with a low dry matter like fresh grass contains a lot of water, and each mouthful the horse takes contains relatively few nutrients, so that the horse has to eat a large amount of it.

Further tests are then carried out on the dried food to discover the protein, energy, fibre and oil content of the dry matter.

**Table 4.1**  Approximate bodyweights.

| Height (hh) | Type | Weight (kg) | Weight (lb) |
|---|---|---|---|
| 10 | pony | 200 | 440 |
| 12.2 | pony | 300 | 660 |
| 13 | pony | 350 | 770 |
| 13 | foal/weanling | 200 | 440 |
| 14 | pony or yearling | 400 | 880 |
| 14.2 | pony | 450 | 990 |
| 14.2 | cob | 500 | 1100 |
| 15 | hack | 450 | 990 |
| 16 | thoroughbred | 550 | 1210 |
| 16 | hunter | 600 | 1320 |
| 16.2 | hunter | 650 | 1430 |
| 17 | shire | 1000 | 2200 |

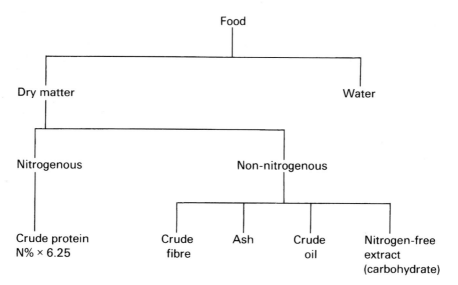

**Fig. 4.2**  The protein makeup of food.

# Measuring energy

The majority of feedstuffs fed to horses consist of a mixture of nutrients: carbohydrate, protein, vitamins, minerals and water. The energy from a feed is derived from various sources including starch, sugar and fibre. Some of these energy sources are more digestible than others. In the laboratory the feed can be tested to discover how much energy it contains and how much is digestible.

The gross energy of the food is the total energy contained within the feed, and is measured as the heat given off when the feed is burned in a calorimeter. Obviously not all of this energy is available to the horse; no feed is 100 per cent digestible otherwise the horse would never produce any droppings. The energy lost in the faeces can be measured and subtracted from the gross energy to give a measure of how much of that energy is actually digestible – the digestible energy (DE). In addition the horse loses energy from the feed through the urine and gases produced internally; the digestible energy minus the energy lost this way gives the metabolisable energy – the energy available for the horse's metabolic processes such as tissue repair, muscle contraction, milk production etc. The efficiency with which the horse's body uses this energy depends on the type of feed: for example, fibrous feeds are not broken down and used as efficiently as starchy feeds, resulting in a larger amount of heat being given off during their digestion and assimilation – feeding forage helps keep the horse warm during winter. This heat loss is known as the heat increment, leaving behind the net energy which is used for growth, work, reproduction and maintenance.

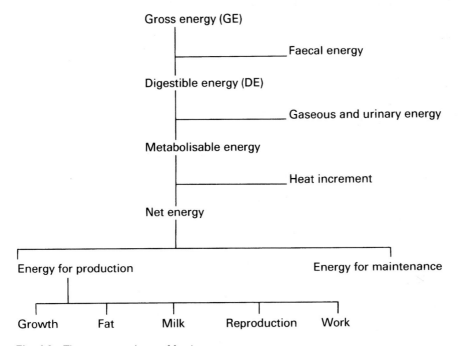

**Fig. 4.3**  The energy makeup of food.

A non-working, stabled horse that is maintaining a stable bodyweight is satisfying its energy requirements for maintenance; this is the basic energy requirement that further rations are built on.

## Calorie counting for horses

The energy part of the horse's ration can be measured, just as anyone who has been on a diet has measured the energy in his or her own food. Once we know the energy in the feedstuffs we can feed exactly the right quantities of feed to satisfy the horse's energy requirements, avoiding overfeeding with its associated metabolic and behavioural problems, or underfeeding and a loss of performance.

Many human feeds now declare the nutrient content on the package. The energy content is stated as both the calorie content and the number of kilojoules present; joules are metric calories. We are all familiar with the principle of dieting, rationing ourselves to a certain number of calories a day, counting the calories in the food and consequently losing weight. We can calorie count for our horses just as we do for ourselves, and this concept is the basis of correct rationing.

Many compound feed manufacturers will publish the energy content of their feeds and tables of approximate energy values are available. Hay can be analysed so that you can allow for its contribution to the energy part of the horse's requirements. Horse feed energy values are usually given as megajoules (multiples of 1 000 000 joules) of digestible energy per kilogram.

## Heat production

Waste heat is a measure of the efficiency of utilisation of the metabolisable energy (ME) of the food and varies between types of feed. In a cold environment heat production is a bonus, while, for the performance horse

**Table 4.2**   Energy values of some common horse feeds.

| Feed | Digestible energy MJ per kg dry matter | Digestible energy MJ per 'scoop' (2 litres) |
|---|---|---|
| Oats | 11–12 | 10 |
| Barley | 13 | 15 |
| Maize | 14 | 19 |
| Extracted soyabean meal | 13.3 | 17 |
| Wheatbran | 11 | 5 |

working in hot conditions, heat production is a disadvantage. Thus the feed chosen for a horse should reflect the climate and the work the horse is doing. Allowance for this is the basis of the French (INRA) Net Energy (NE) system. Estimates of the efficiency of ME utilisation show that 30 per cent of the energy of meadow hay is lost as heat but only 15 per cent of the ME of barley would be lost. This indicates that hay is a useful feed for outwintered horses in cold weather as it helps keep them warm. Excess waste heat in working horses is a hindrance, thus concentrate feeds not only supply the high energy demands of the performance horse, but also help reduce heat stress.

## Measuring protein

Proteins consist of long chains of nitrogen-containing amino acids. Laboratory analysis of the protein content of a feed involves measuring the total amount of nitrogen present by the Kjeldhal method. Once the amount of nitrogen has been determined the percentage of crude protein is calculated. The crude protein overestimates the protein available to the horse because, firstly, not all the crude protein is digestible and secondly, not all the nitrogen present in a feed is present as protein. There are other non-protein nitrogen substances present such as urea, nitrates and ammonia, which are not as valuable to the horse as amino acids.

The digestible crude protein (DCP) gives an indication of the protein actually available to the horse and is much more useful for designing rations. Unfortunately much of the work done to determine the digestibility of different protein sources has been done on animals other than

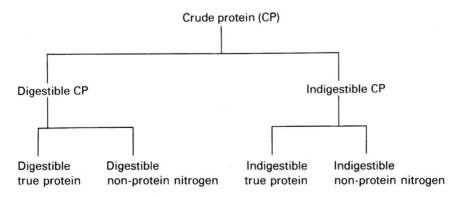

**Fig. 4.4** Estimating the protein in food.

horses. The result is that you may see the 'estimated DCP' on a feed bag, the estimation having used information from other animals.

Remember too, that the quality of the protein in terms of its essential amino acid composition is very important in equine nutrition.

# The energy requirements for maintenance

The energy requirements for maintenance are those resulting in no weight change in a stabled, resting horse. An idle horse obviously has relatively low energy requirements, but its appetite should be satisfied to avoid the horse getting bored and developing stable vices. Bulky fibrous feeds contain less energy per kilogram dry matter, so the horse has to eat more to satisfy its requirements.

Many workers have estimated the horse's maintenance requirements, coming up with varying results. The major reason for the variation is that, unlike other animals, horses cannot be closely confined; they need a certain amount of exercise, even if only moving around in a large stable. The amount of exercise and the type of horse used will affect the maintenance requirement results.

The horse's maintenance requirements are related to the horse's bodyweight and are usually expressed as the requirements per 100 kg bodyweight. A simple relationship of 12.5 MJ of DE per 100 kg bodyweight per day gives the maintenance requirement of a 16 hh horse on box rest after injury or illness; it only needs 8–9 kg (17–20 lb) of hay a day to satisfy all its energy requirements.

The horse's maintenance requirement under practical conditions is most affected by the climate. The horse, like the human being, is a warm-

**Table 4.3**  The relationship between height, bodyweight and maintenance requirement.

| Height (hh) | Bodyweight (kg) | Mainenance requirement (MJ DE/day) | Ration (kg/day hay at 8 MJ DE/kg) |
|---|---|---|---|
| 11 | 200–260 | 25–32.5 | 3–4 |
| 12 | 230–290 | 29–36 | 3.6–4.5 |
| 13 | 290–350 | 36–44 | 4.5–5.5 |
| 14 | 350–420 | 44–52.5 | 5.5–6.5 |
| 15 | 420–520 | 52.5–65 | 6.5–8 |
| 16 | 500–600 | 62.5–75 | 8–9 |
| 17 | 600–725 | 75–90 | 9–11 |

blooded animal designed to keep its body temperature greater than that of its surroundings; this means that heat is continually being lost. In cold, wet or windy conditions the horse's metabolic rate increases so that the rate of heat production keeps pace with the increased rate of heat loss and the horse can thus maintain a steady body temperature. This in turn means that the horse's maintenance requirements increase. In hot weather the horse's metabolic rate will slow down to minimise heat production and the maintenance requirement for energy will fall.

Fibrous feeds like hay, which are not digested as efficiently as concentrate feeds, result in more heat being produced, and this 'warming' effect may be very useful for horses at grass in winter. This effect may not be so beneficial in horses in hard work which have higher energy requirements; poor quality roughages are an expensive buy if they form a major part of the ration of hard-working or growing horses and may result in loss of condition.

## The protein requirements for maintenance

The adult horse needs a maintenance level of protein in the diet to supply the amino acids necessary to replace body tissue, enzymes, hair and skin that is lost due to normal wear and tear. The energy requirement of the resting horse is such that if the energy requirement is satisfied, then the protein requirement will also be catered for – look after the energy and the protein will look after itself.

The horse at rest needs 7.5–8 per cent crude protein in the ration. A diet of good quality hay will supply adequate energy and protein levels; however if the hay is of dubious quality, the hay ration may need to be supplemented to raise the protein level. Care must be taken not to overfeed the horse at rest; if concentrates have to be introduced, the hay may need to be rationed.

## The energy requirements for work

Working horses have to convert the energy gained from their feed into muscle power for disciplines as varied as endurance riding and flat racing, and diets must be formulated to reflect these different needs. Correct feeding is an essential and integral part of the horse's training programme.

**Table 4.4**  Nutrient values of common feeds.

| | Crude protein (%) | Digestible energy (MJ DE/kg) | | Crude protein (%) | Digestible energy (MJ DE/kg) |
|---|---|---|---|---|---|
| Hay | | | Barley | 9.5 | 13 |
| *Average* | 4.5–8 | 7–8 | Maize | 8.5 | 14 |
| *Good* | 9–10 | 9 | Linseed | 22 | 18.5 |
| *Poor* | 3.5–6 | 7 | Extracted | | |
| Silage | | | soyabean meal | 44 | 13.3 |
| *Clamp* | 11 | 9–10 | Peas | 23 | 14 |
| *Big bale* | 10 | 10 | Grassmeal | 16 | 9.6 |
| Haylage | 9–12 | 9–11.5 | Alfalfa meal | 17 | 9 |
| Straw | 3 | 6 | Wheatbran | 15.5 | 11 |
| Oats | 9.6 | 11–12 | Sugar beet pulp | 7 | 110.5 |
| Naked oats | 13.5 | 16 | Vegetable oil | 0 | 35 |
| | | | Molasses | 3 | 11 |

The energy requirements for work depend on many factors including

- speed of the work
- duration of the work
- terrain
- incline
- the weight of the horse
- the horse's fitness
- rider/driver ability
- environmental temperature and humidity
- the horse's soundness and conformation.

At one extreme a sprint race of six furlongs theoretically increases a horse's daily energy requirements by a mere 4 per cent, while a day's hunting would more than double the day's energy requirement. In sprint races the majority of the energy for muscle contraction is obtained by the anaerobic breakdown of glucose, whereas long distance horses like eventers, hunters and endurance horses, use a combination of anaerobic and aerobic energy production, where glucose is burnt up in the presence of oxygen to produce the energy for prolonged muscle contraction.

Training involves priming the horse's body systems so that the horse can do the work demanded of it with maximum efficiency and minimum fatigue.

Walking, which is generally accepted to be an extremely good form of exercise for toning muscles, tendons and ligaments, barely increases the horse's daily energy requirement above maintenance. Strenuous or

**Table 4.5**  Digestible energy (DE) demands of maintenance and work.

| Bodyweight (kg) | 200 | 400 | 600 |
| --- | --- | --- | --- |
| Maintenance requirement/day (MJ DE) | 35 | 58 | 79 |
| *Energy requirement for work: (MJ DE/day)* | | | |
| 1 hour walking | 0.4 | 0.8 | 1.3 |
| 1 hour slow trotting, some cantering | 4.2 | 8.4 | 12.5 |
| 1 hour fast trotting, cantering, some jumping | 10.5 | 20.9 | 31 |
| Cantering, galloping and jumping | 25 | 50 | 75 |
| Strenuous, effort, racing, polo | 42.0 | 85 | 127 |
| Endurance work, 100 km in 10.5 hours | 43.5 | 87 | 130.5 |

extended effort increases the horse's requirement to such an extent that the horse physically cannot eat that much energy in one day; thus recovery from hard work requires several days for the horse's energy reserves to be replenished.

Experiments on horses and ponies working on treadmills with an incline show that working uphill increases the energy requirement 17 times. Work over uneven and hilly ground is much more arduous than on flat terrain.

Even though during hard work a horse will use up more energy than he can consume during the day, we must not feed him to fortify him for future events, because any energy supplied over and above immediate needs will be stored as fat, and fatness will impair performance. Overfeeding can also lead to problems such as filled legs, laminitis, colic, azoturia and excitability.

## The protein requirements for work

The horse's dietary requirement for protein is not greatly increased by work. The loss of protein in sweat, and the protein incorporated into the greater muscle mass of the fit horse is reflected by an increase of about 2 per cent in the diet. As the horse works, the energy requirement increases substantially; the concentrate ration fed to sustain this energy require-

**Table 4.6**  The protein needed for different types of work.

| Work level | Crude protein in the ration (%) |
| --- | --- |
| Light | 7.5–8 |
| Medium | 7.5–8 |
| Hard | 9.5–10 |
| Fast | 9.5–10 |

ment very often increases the protein component of the ration sufficiently to meet the extra protein demand.

The feeding of excess protein may in fact, be detrimental to performance with horses not racing as fast and sweating and blowing more heavily. Horses with high energy requirements do not need to be fed high protein feeds, unless they are being fed extremely poor hay, with a protein content of below 6 per cent.

The exception to these statements are two and three-year-old racehorses in training, which are still growing and consequently have a high protein requirement.

## The energy requirements for pregnancy

The mare is pregnant for approximately 11 months; her dietary requirements can be divided into two periods, the first eight months of pregnancy and the last three months.

### The first eight months

The foetus undergoes tremendous developmental changes during the first eight months of the gestation period but makes very little growth. The minimal growth of the foetus makes no practical impact on the mare's energy requirements. This means that up until Christmas, if she is in good condition, the mare should be treated no differently from a barren mare in terms of her feed. A mare with a foal at foot will already be receiving extra feed to provide for lactation, and pregnancy will not increase this requirement. After weaning, a mare in good condition can just be fed for maintenance until the last three months of her pregnancy.

### The last 90 days

Most of the growth of the foetus takes place during the last 90 days of pregnancy and consequently the mare's energy requirement increases. The extra energy needed by the mare is surprisingly low, amounting to approximately 6 per cent of her maintenance requirement, which is equivalent in energy terms to the mare doing light work.

## The protein requirements for pregnancy

The most critical nutrients for breeding mares given traditional feeds are protein, calcium and phosphorus; these are laid down in large amounts in the tissue of the developing foetus. Like the energy requirement, the protein requirement only increases significantly in the last 90 days of pregnancy. The mare in the first eight months of pregnancy is fed for maintenance (8 per cent crude protein); in the last 90 days her requirement increases to 10 per cent. It is unlikely that even good quality hay will supply 10 per cent protein and supplementary protein will be needed. If the hay contains 7 per cent protein and the mare is receiving a ratio of 70:30, hay to concentrates, the concentrate must be at least 16 per cent crude protein to make up the shortfall of the hay.

## The energy requirements for lactation

The amount of energy a mare requires for lactation will depend on how much milk she produces (i.e. how much the foal drinks) and the composition of the milk. It has been estimated that a mare can produce up to 5 per cent of her bodyweight of milk a day; this is equivalent to a 500 kg mare producing 25 kg or 5.5 gallons per day. This is a high figure and will be limited by the foal's appetite. However foals suckle frequently, up to 100 times a day in the first week, and the mare's udders rarely look full, leading to the impression that she is not producing much milk.

There is no doubt that the energy requirement for lactation is much greater than for pregnancy, amounting to 15 times that for gestation in total. This gives the lactating brood mare a daily energy requirement approximating to that of a horse in medium to hard work; i.e. a 500 kg mare will need an extra 50 MJ DE per day on top of her maintenance requirement.

The calcium and phosphorus needed for milk production substantially increase the mare's need for these two minerals.

## The protein requirements for lactation

There is little difference between breeds or individuals in the composition of mare's milk; in all cases the composition changes rapidly during the first days of lactation. The first milk that the mare produces is called colostrum, which is high in immunoglobulins (antibodies), dry matter and vitamin A. The antibodies pass on a degree of passive immunity to the foal so that it is protected against infection until its own immune system is beginning to function.

The protein content of the mare's milk is around 19 per cent for 30 minutes after giving birth; by 12 hours this drops to about 4 per cent and by eight days falls to a fairly steady 2 per cent. This changing protein level means that the mare's requirement for dietary protein will also change, but it is not practical to change the mare's feed frequently. Instead average values are taken for the two halves of her lactation, assuming that the foal will be weaned at six to seven months. The lactating mare will need 12.5 per cent crude protein in the ration in the first three months. Subsequently she will need 11 per cent crude protein.

## The energy requirements for growth

The way in which animals grow is complex; they do not just get bigger and heavier, the organs and tissues of the body also develop. Newly-born foals grow very rapidly, and the rate of growth declines as the horse approaches maturity. The trends in growth and development determine the young horse's requirements for energy, protein, minerals and vitamins.

As a rough guide, a Thoroughbred foal's birthweight is about 10 per cent of its adult weight. Birthweight is very important in determining the horse's ultimate mature weight, and foals weighing less than 35 kg are unlikely to make more than 15 hh. Birthweight is affected by several factors including:

- nutrition of the mare
- the uterine environment
- age of the mare
- sex of the foal
- time of year born – later foals tend to be heavier and taller.

**Table 4.7**  Percentage of mature bodyweight and withers height attained at various ages.*

| Age | 6 months | | 12 months | | 18 months | |
|---|---|---|---|---|---|---|
| | Weight | Height | Weight | Height | Weight | Height |
| Shetland pony | 52 | 86 | 73 | 94 | 83 | 97 |
| Quarter horse | 44 | 84 | 66 | 91 | 80 | 95 |
| Anglo-Arab | 45 | 83 | 67 | 92 | 81 | 95 |
| Arab | 46 | 84 | 66 | 91 | 80 | 95 |
| Thoroughbred | 46 | 84 | 66 | 90 | 80 | 95 |
| Percheron | 40 | 79 | 59 | 89 | 74 | 92 |

*From Hintz, 1980

The young horse should achieve 60–70 per cent of its mature weight and about 90 per cent of its mature height by the time it is 12 months old, providing that it has received adequate nutrition. The time of weaning should not affect this if the management before and after weaning has been good.

Bone is the earliest maturing tissue and a horse's ultimate height is determined in very early life. This means that the young foal demands a diet rich in bone-forming minerals, vitamins and protein. As the foal's growth rate slows down and it begins to lay down muscle and finally fat, it requires more carbohydrate in the diet. Horses or ponies receiving a slightly less than adequate diet will still reach the same mature size as those that are well fed; however they will take longer to attain their mature height and weight. Those on severely limited rations may never reach their full potential, due to abnormal growth and development of the skeleton.

Agricultural animals grown for meat are encouraged to grow as quickly as possible; this is not without risk in horses, and the best pattern of growth for optimum athletic performance is not known. The racing two-year-old Thoroughbred is grown very quickly and experiences growth-related problems, such as developmental orthopaedic diseases (DOD) which are discussed in Chapter 7. Generally speaking the growth curve should be as smooth as possible.

It is possible to estimate the energy in each kilogram of bodyweight that a foal gains, and work out a ration that satisfies this requirement, but this is retrospective and not very practical. From weaning until the flush of spring grass the following year, youngstock should receive 1.25–1.6 kg of

**Table 4.8** The relationship between bodyweight and withers height in normally growing horses.

| Breed | Height (hh) | Weight (kg) | Age |
|-------|-------------|-------------|-----|
| Pony | 9 | 60 | 2 months |
| | 10 | 80 | 4 months |
| | 11.2 | 140 | 9 months |
| | 12 | 180 | 12 months |
| | 13 | 320 (mature) | 3 years |
| Thoroughbred | 10 | 50 | Birth |
| | 11 | 90 | 6–8 weeks |
| | 12 | 140 | 8–12 weeks |
| | 13 | 200 | 4–6 months |
| | 14.2 | 350 | 9–12 months |
| | 15.2 | 450 (mature) | 2–3 years |

**Table 4.9**   Daily feed allowances for horses expected to reach 500 kg mature weight (15.2–16 hh).

| Bodyweight (kg) | Concentrates (kg) | Concentrates (lb) | Hay (kg) | Hay (lb) |
|---|---|---|---|---|
| *Foals* | | | | |
| 80 (4-5 weeks) | 0.5 | 1 | – | – |
| 130–180 (8–12 weeks) | 2.2–3.2 | 5–7 | 1.3–1.9 | 3–4 |
| 180–230 (2–4 months) | 2.9–3.9 | 6–8 | 1.8–2.3 | 4–5 |
| 230–270 (4–6 months) | 3.6–4.8 | 8–10 | 2.2–2.8 | 5–6 |
| 270–320 (6–8 months) | 4–4.6 | 9–10 | 2.7–3.2 | 6–7 |
| *Yearlings* | | | | |
| 310–360 (8–10 months) | 3.5–4.5 | 8–10 | 3–3.7 | 7–8 |
| 360–410 (10–12 months) | 3.0–4.2 | 7–9 | 3.6–4.1 | 8–9 |
| 410–460 (12–14 months) | 3–3.8 | 7–8 | 4–4.5 | 9–10 |

concentrates per 100 kg bodyweight (16 per cent crude protein), with appropriate mineral and vitamin supplementation.

This means that a Thoroughbred weanling about 13 hh, weighing 200 kg will receive 2.5–3.2 kg of concentrate feed a day. As the youngster grows during the winter its concentrate ration increases to 4.5 kg. Once the yearling has attained 90 per cent of its mature bodyweight, usually when going into its second winter as a long yearling, it should be fed for maintenance, as a mature horse, unless it is to be raced as a two-year-old or produced for the show ring.

## The protein requirements for growth

A young horse with an expected mature weight of 450–500 kg would normally gain 100 kg of bodyweight between the ages of 3 and 6 months; this is equivalent to about 1 kg per day. The next 100 kg is gained by the time it is 12 months old (0.5 kg/day), and the remaining weight slowly acquired until the horse reaches its mature weight.

The rate of growth of bone and muscle, and hence the protein requirement, is most rapid in the foal, and gradually slows down as the horse approaches maturity. The quality of the protein given to young horses is very important; the essential amino acid lysine, which is frequently lacking in horse diets, is particularly important. Thoroughbred yearlings have a lysine requirement of 4.5 g lysine per kg of total diet. As the lysine present in cereals and hay is very variable, any stud ration should contain at least 7 g lysine per kg. If a ration based on oats and hay is being fed the youngster will need a supplement which will supply 20 g of lysine.

The lysine levels in grass are also variable; using cereals to supplement the young horse's diet may mean that the lysine requirement is not met and a suitable supplement should be used.

## The nutrient requirements of stallions

The feeding of stallions is surrounded by mystery; the extra nutrients needed for sperm production are very small and there is no evidence that using special supplements will enhance sperm production and fertility. During the winter the resting stallion should be fed like any other horse with a maintenance ration of clean hay supplemented with a low energy concentrate such as a horse and pony cube. If the stallion works or competes he would be fed for that work with a correctly balanced ration. During the covering season the stallion's energy requirements increase as he is used for teasing and covering. While the energy expended may not be great compared to galloping and jumping, many stallions fret, pacing their stables and losing condition. Large quantities of concentrate feeds are not desirable (indeed many horses will refuse to eat large amounts of hard feed), so good quality forage is essential. Haylage or top-quality hay may tempt him to eat and help maintain condition.

If the stallion is in good condition, do not feel compelled to give him concentrates; providing he is receiving a balanced ration it is better to keep him fit not fat.

## The NE system

*Energy*

Firstly, the NE system expresses the Net Energy (NE) content of feedstuffs for maintenance, expressed in UFCs; 1UFC is equivalent to 9.414 MJ NE.

The NE content of feeds for maintenance is calculated from their ME value, taking into account how efficiently the feed is utilised. Table 4.10 compares DE and NE values for commonly fed concentrates and forages.

Table 4.10    Comparison of the DE and NE values for concentrates and forages.

|  | DE (MJ/kg) | UFC* |
| --- | --- | --- |
| Barley | 15.2 | 1.163 |
| Maize | 16.1 | 1.35 |
| Oats | 13.4 | 1.01 |
| Grass hay | 7.3 | 0.53 |
| Barley straw | 6.8 | 0.28 |

*UFC = Unité Fourragère Cheval

### Protein

The scheme also accounts for the digestible crude protein (DCP) of feeds. The useful protein is calculated from the estimated quantity of amino acids absorbed from the gut and is measured as MADC (g/kg DM).

Table 4.11    Digestible crude protein values compared to MADC.

|  | DCP (g) | MADC* (g) |
| --- | --- | --- |
| Spring grass | 128 | 117 |
| Barley | 90 | 90 |
| Grass hay | 65 | 54 |

*MADC = Matières Azotées Digestibles Corrigées (or Cheval)

### Maintenance

The energy maintenance requirement is calculated as:

$$0.038 \text{ UFC/kg BW}^{0.75}$$

or

4 UFC/day for an adult 500 kg gelding.

The daily protein requirement for maintenance of an adult horse is:

$$2.8 \text{ g MADC/kg BW}^{0.75}$$

or

295 g MADC/day for a 500 kg horse.

**Table 4.12**   Daily energy (UFC) and protein (MADC) requirements of horses as proposed by INRA.*

| Adult weight (kg) | 450 | | 500 | | 600 | |
|---|---|---|---|---|---|---|
| | UFC | MADC | UFC | MADC | UFC | MADC |
| Maintenance | 3.9 | 275 | 4.2 | 295 | 4.8 | 340 |
| Light work | 6.6 | 450 | 6.9 | 470 | 7.5 | 510 |
| Medium works[1] | 7.6 | 515 | 7.9 | 540 | 8.5 | 580 |
| Intense work[2] | 6.9 | 470 | 7.2 | 490 | 7.8 | 530 |
| *Mare, gestation* | | | | | | |
| Month 8 | 3.8 | 315 | 4.1 | 340 | 4.7 | 395 |
| Months 9–10 | 4.3 | 425 | 4.7 | 460 | 5.4 | 535 |
| Month 11 | 4.4 | 445 | 4.8 | 485 | 5.5 | 565 |
| *Mare, lactation* | | | | | | |
| Month 1 | 8.2 | 865 | 8.9 | 950 | 10.5 | 1125 |
| Month 2 | 7.0 | 700 | 7.6 | 770 | 8.9 | 910 |
| Month 3 | 7.0 | 700 | 7.6 | 770 | 8.9 | 910 |
| *Growth* | | | | | | |
| 6 months | 4.2 | 500 | 4.5 | 530 | 5.1 | 600 |
| 8–12 months | 5.1 | 560 | 5.5 | 590 | 6.2 | 660 |
| 20–24 months | 6.3 | 380 | 6.8 | 420 | 7.8 | 660 |
| 32–36 months | 5.9 | 300 | 6.5 | 330 | 7.6 | 390 |
| *Stallion[3]* | | | | | | |
| Resting | 5.8 | 400 | 6.1 | 420 | 6.3 | 440 |
| Breeding | 6.6–8 | 480–620 | 7.0–8.4 | 490–630 | 7.0–8.5 | 520–650 |

*Anon 1984, updated by INRA, Ed Martin-Rosset 1990
[1] 2 hour daily
[2] 1 hour daily
[3] 0.5 hours exercise daily

# The nutrient requirements of old age

As horses age they seem to have less resistance to cold weather, worms, viruses and skin diseases. Just as in humans the ageing process is a gradual one, some horses will feel old at 12 years of age, while others are fine at the age of 20, or even older. Older horses need to be fed and looked after carefully if they are to continue working happily or to enjoy a healthy and contented retirement. Many old horses have lost some of their teeth or have sharp teeth, which reduces their ability to chew hay, grains and cubes. Pain and discomfort from arthritis may stop the horse moving around and grazing freely, as well as possibly reducing his appetite. As horses age their digestive efficiency decreases and they need more energy for everyday life. Older horses also need higher levels of good quality protein as well as higher levels of calcium and phosphorus in their rations.

To help him keep his condition the older horse's diet needs to be:

- very tasty
- easy to eat, and
- rich in nutrients.

Most feed manufacturers make mixes specially for veteran horses and ponies which are rich in energy and protein and contain higher levels of minerals and vitamins. These feeds are usually highly palatable soft mixes which are easy to eat. The majority of manufacturers design these feeds to be compatible with others in their range; veteran or conditioning feed may make up all or just part of the concentrate ration, depending on the horse's individual requirements.

## Nutrition of the sick horse

Providing the horse with a balanced ration plays an important part in the horse's ability to fight illness, and correct nutrition provides one of the body's defence mechanisms. Proper feeding of the sick horse should always be considered as an integral part of the sick nursing and the therapeutic regime.

The task of feeding the sick horse can be difficult and tiresome; the horse's appetite is likely to be depressed, swallowing may be difficult and the function of the gut may be disturbed. Any upset in gut function may lead to dehydration and a disturbance of the electrolyte balance, occurring just when the horse's metabolic requirements may be substantially greater. This means that there is often marked weight loss during illness, with a resultant decrease in the horse's defence capacity, prolonging illness and convalescence.

The treatment of illness is aimed at removing the cause of the illness or injury and also the removal of any damaged tissue. Controlled nutritional management is helpful in breaking the cycle of disease; it can minimise body tissue wastage and reduce the after-effects of the illness so that convalescence is reduced.

### The metabolic effects of disease

Although this has not been extensively studied in horses, in humans a fever raises the metabolic rate 13 per cent for every 1°C of temperature rise. If one assumes that a similar situation arises in horses, then trauma will increase the metabolic rate by over 25 per cent. Sometimes a horse will compensate for this by eating more, but sick horses usually go off their feed and the horse loses condition. This loss of condition is associated with a drop in the efficiency of the immune system and a vicious circle is set up.

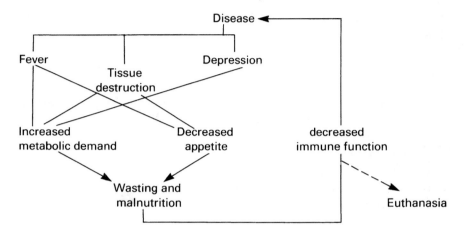

**Fig. 4.5**   The circle of disease.

## Diets for the sick horse

The sick horse's diet must have several special characteristics:

- palatability
- good quality protein
- fibre
- minerals and vitamins.

### Palatibility

The horse must be provided with the most palatable feed possible to encourage it to eat. Barn-dried hay is ideal if the horse has previously been fed poor quality hay. Maize can be gradually introduced into the diet; it is acceptable and has a high energy content. Molasses, mashes and succulents can all be used providing that the food is fresh. If swallowing is difficult the feeds should be soft and any succulent cut into very small pieces. If chewing is a problem the horse may need a liquid diet.

Little and often is vital for the sick horse, with up to eight feeds a day, including first thing in the morning and last thing at night. Any rejected food should be cleared out immediately. Soaking or damping hay may help, and will also mean that the horse is taking in water. A smear of vapour rub in the false nostril may mask the smell of medicines in the feed.

Plenty of fresh clean water must always be available, and it should be changed frequently. If the horse is using an automatic drinking system, close it off and give the water by bucket so that you can monitor the amount the horse drinks.

## Protein content

The protein content of the sick horse's diet is more important than the amount of energy, because the horse is not active and protein is needed for the repair of body tissue. Underfeeding may even delay healing and depress the efficiency of the immune system. Good quality grass nuts, milk pellets, stud cubes and soyabean meal are all high in good quality protein. While adult horses cannot utilise the milk sugar, milk pellets have the advantage of being a highly palatable source of good protein.

## Fibre content

Fibre is important in maintaining normal gut function: it binds the food residue together as faeces and aids proper elimination of the faeces. As the fibre content of the diet increases, so its digestibility falls and a compromise has to be reached. Molassed sugar beet pulp and bran are useful palatable sources of fibre and can be fed as mashes.

## Minerals and vitamins

The sick horse may become severely dehydrated and it is important to supply a suitable source of electrolytes to help restore the fluid balance of the body. A supplement of minerals/vitamins/amino acids may be recommended by the vet, depending on the horse's blood profile. An anaemic horse would require iron, folic acid and vitamin $B_{12}$ as well as a normal broad spectrum supplement. As always, limestone and salt are important.

# Chapter 5
# Ration Formulation

A balanced ration provides energy, protein, minerals, vitamins and water in sufficient quantities to keep the horse alive and allow it to do the work we demand. The nutrient demands of a horse will depend on many factors including:

- size
- appetite
- condition
- work done
- age

- reproductive status
- health
- environment
- management.

The amount of nutrients a horse needs and the amount that it can consume are dependent on its size, and more specifically, its bodyweight. As discussed in Chapter 4 there are several methods of determining the horse's bodyweight; Table 5.1 illustrates approximate bodyweights and appetites for different horses and ponies.

This value for bodyweight can now be used as a basis for calculating energy requirements and appetite. Generally a horse will eat about 2.5 per cent of his bodyweight per day; growing foals and lactating broodmares

Table 5.1 The relationship between height, girth, bodyweight and appetite.

| Height (hh) | Girth (cm) | Bodyweight (kg) | Appetite (kg dry matter) |
|---|---|---|---|
| 11 | 135–145 | 200–260 | 4.5–6 |
| 12 | 140–150 | 230–290 | 5–7 |
| 13 | 150–160 | 290–350 | 6.5–8 |
| 14 | 160–170 | 350–420 | 8–9.5 |
| 15 | 170–185 | 420–520 | 10–12.5 |
| 16 | 185–195 | 500–600 | 12–14 |
| 17 | 195–210 | 600–725 | 13–18 |

NB: The values in this table are averages and only approximate have high nutrient requirements and may eat more than this. For example, a 15.2 hh horse weighing 500 kg will be able to eat a maximum of 12.5 kg dry matter per day and any ration we design must allow for this; it is no good creating a balanced, palatable ration if the horse physically cannot eat it all. This is the amount of dry matter a horse can eat in a day; obviously he will eat a much greater weight of grass, which is 75 per cent water, than he will of hay, which is only 15 per cent water.

## Condition

One of the first things anybody notices about a horse, regardless of size or type, is its condition – is it fat or thin? If it is thin then the nutrient requirement for energy will be higher to enable it to put on condition. Assessment of condition is very subjective, and care must be taken to look at the whole picture, because while a show horse would look fat in a racing yard, a racehorse would look very lean in a showing yard. The type and intensity of work that the horse is doing must also be taken into consideration.

Condition can be assessed objectively using a method originally designed for farm livestock, called condition scoring. Condition is measured using a scoring system from 0 to 5, assessing manually and visually the horse's weight displacement along the neck, over the back ribs and over the quarters (Fig. 5.1).

To condition score a horse stand directly behind it and note the amount of flesh covering the pelvis and top of the quarters, the flanks and beneath the tail. Assess the tautness of skin over the pelvis and compare your findings to the comments in Table 5.2. The backbone and ribs are scored by observing and feeling the horse from both sides. Finally the neck is scored by standing by the horse's shoulder and noting the shape and feel of the neck just in front of the withers.

A horse with a condition score of 0 is starving, with sharp and prominent croup and hip bones, cut up behind and with a prominent rib-cage. A thin horse would have a condition score of 1: the bones are still prominent but there is more muscle definition. Horses with a score of 2 are approaching normal: the hip bones and vertebrae of the back are defined but not prominent, as would be expected in fit horses such as hunters and eventers. Those with a score of 3 are getting fat and the bones become more difficult to feel as one would expect with a horse in show condition. Scores 4 and 5 indicate obesity, with large masses of fat on the neck, quarters and back. The ribs can only be felt on pressure.

| Condition score | Back | Pelvis | Comment |
|---|---|---|---|
| 4 | 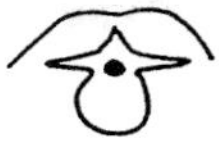 | 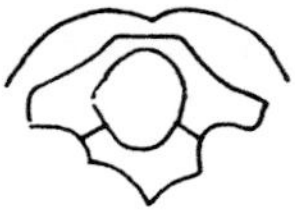 | **Obese:** Large masses of fat carried on neck quarters and back. Can only feel ribs on pressure. |
| 3 | 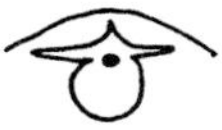 | 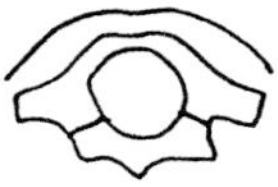 | **Getting fat:** Bones becoming more difficult to feel. *Show horses.* |
| 2 | 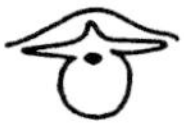 | 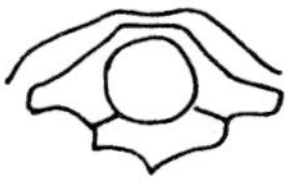 | **Approaching normal:** Hip bones and vertebrae of back defined but not prominent. *Hunters & eventers.* |
| 1 | 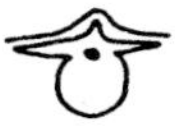 | 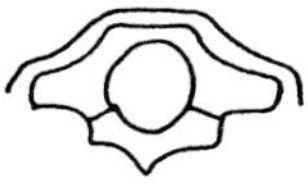 | **Thin:** Bones still prominent but a little more muscle definition. |
| 0 | 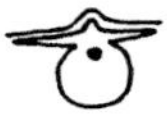 | 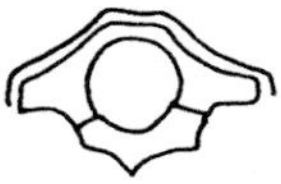 | **Starvation:** Croup and hip bones sharp and prominent. Cut-up behind. Rib cage prominent. |

**Fig. 5.1**  Condition scoring.

## Skin and coat condition

The coat should be glossy and feel smooth and silky; the skin should be loose and pliable and when picked up in a pinch and released it should return smoothly and easily to its former position. Any delay indicates either a degree of dehydration or a lack of subcutaneous fat.

## Blood testing

Blood testing assesses the horse's internal condition; sub-clinical illness which causes below-par performance may only be detected through blood testing. The problem may be worms, bacterial or viral infection, dehydration or anaemia. Occasionally a change in diet may be all that is needed, or it may be a job for the vet. A blood test every four to six months can be an invaluable tool to help you feed your horse and get it fit.

**Table 5.2**  Condition scoring.

| Condition Score | Pelvis | Back and ribs | Base of neck |
| --- | --- | --- | --- |
| 0 | Deep cavity under tail and either side of croup. Pelvis angular. No detectable fatty tissue between skin and bone. | Processes of vertebrae sharp to touch. Skin drawn tightly over ribs. | Ewe neck, very narrow and slack at base. |
| 1 | Pelvis and croup well defined, no fatty tissue but skin supple. Poverty lines visible and deep depression under tail. | Ribs and backbone clearly defined but skin slack over the bones. | Ewe neck, narrow and slack at base. |
| 2 | Croup well defined but some fatty tissue under skin. Pelvis easily felt, slight depression under tail. | Backbone just covered by fatty tissue, individual processes not visible but easily felt on pressure. Ribs just visible. | Narrow but firm. |
| 3 | Whole pelvic region rounded, not angular and no 'gutter' along croup. Skin smooth and supple, pelvis easily felt. | Backbone and ribs well covered but easily felt on pressure. | Narrow but with no crest except for stallions. |
| 4 | Pelvis buried in fatty tissue and only felt on firm pressure. Gutter over croup. | Backbone and ribs well covered and only felt on firm pressure. Gutter along backbone. | Wide and firm with folds of fatty tissue, slight crest even in mares. |
| 5 | Pelvis buried in firm fatty tissue and cannot be felt. Clear deep gutter over croup to base of dock. Skin stretched. | Back looks flat with deep gutter along backbone. Ribs buried and cannot be felt. | Very wide and firm, marked crest, even in mares. |

## Tooth condition

A tooth problem can make a horse difficult to ride and cause him to lose condition. Do not overlook this simple management check. Teeth must be looked at and rasped regularly – at least twice a year, and as often as every six weeks if the horse has a problem.

## Hoof condition

Dry, flaky and brittle hooves can be an indication that the horse's diet is not balanced, although the effects of shoeing and environment cannot be ignored. If the horse is receiving a good quality diet and looks well in all other respects, the horse may be suffering from a specific shortage of hoof-forming elements. The substances involved in building up and maintaining healthy hoof horn include biotin, sulphur, zinc, lysine and methionine; supplements containing these minerals, vitamins and amino acids are available.

## Work done

One of the old-established rules of feeding is to feed the horse for the amount and intensity of the work it is doing. It is important for the horse's health, your safety and your joint success not to overfeed or underfeed your horse for his degree of fitness. This means that one of the first steps in rationing is to establish the horse's performance or competitive goal in order to get the horse to the correct level of fitness and feeding. There is no point in having a horse, particularly a youngster or a child's pony, too fit and overfed for the task in hand.

## The ratio of forage to concentrates

In the practical situation when a new horse arrives in the yard and you do not know his history, you have to decide what to put on the feedboard immediately and there is no time to get out your calculator. A rule of thumb that has been used for many years to help us decide what to ration horses has been a simple table, relating the intensity of the horse's work to the ratio of forage to concentrate fed (Table 5.3).

**Table 5.3**    The ratio of forage to concentrate for different work levels.

|  | Hay (%) | Concentrates (%) |
|---|---|---|
| Resting | 100 | 0 |
| Light work | 75 | 25 |
| Medium work | 50 | 50 |
| Heavy work | 25 | 75 |

Thus a three-quarterbred horse, of about 16 hh and weighing 500 kg, would be fed as shown in Table 5.4.

**Table 5.4**    Rationing a three-quarterbred horse.

| Height (hh) | Weight kg (lb) | Appetite (2.5% bodyweight) kg (lb) | Work level | Hay | Concentrates |
|---|---|---|---|---|---|
| 15.2–16 | 500 (1100 lb) | 12.5 kg (28 lb) | Resting | 12.5 kg 28 lb | 0 |
|  |  |  | Light | 9 kg 21 lb | 3.5 kg 7 lb |
|  |  |  | Medium | 6.25 kg 14 lb | 6.25 kg 14 lb |
|  |  |  | Heavy | 3.5 kg 7 lb | 9 kg 21 lb |

I do not like the thought of trying to ride a Novice event horse down the centre line of a dressage arena, for example, when it has been fed 14 lb of hard feed. Table 5.5 is revised to give better guidelines:

**Table 5.5**    Revised ratios of forage to concentrates.

| Work level | Hay | Concentrates |
|---|---|---|
| Resting | 100 | 0 |
| Light | 75 | 25 |
| Medium | 60 | 40 |
| Hard | 40 | 60 |
| Fast | 30 | 70 |

This means that our example horse is fed 40 per cent concentrates and 60 per cent forage, resulting in a ration of 5 kg (11 lb) of concentrates and 7.5 kg (17 lb) hay. This may still be too much for many horses but it is much better than before.

Using a guideline like this is useful but has several problems.

*We may not want to feed the horse as much as he can eat*

Horses, like humans, will go off their feed if they are constantly satiated with food. Think of Christmas: you eat as much as you can on Christmas Day and Boxing Day; most of us eat very little on the following days, feeling sick of the sight of food. If you feed a horse as much as it can eat every day, it too will feel like this eventually. It is best to feed a horse slightly below appetite so that he is always eager for his next concentrate feed and has always finished his haynet when you come to fill it again.

Beware of the *ad lib* feeding system: often the hay rack is constantly topped up so that the hay at the bottom becomes mouldy, and the horse becomes over-fussy and wasteful.

If you feed a weighed ration of hay and concentrates, within the horse's appetite, he should always eat up. If he does not eat all his hay and concentrates it may indicate that the quality of the feed is not up to scratch or that the horse is off-colour.

*Which concentrate(s) to feed*

The energy value of different feeds must be considered. A ration composed of a high energy performance cube would make up a smaller proportion of the ration, while low energy horse and pony cubes would need to make up a greater proportion of the ration to meet the same energy demand.

## The rules of rationing

### Step one: estimation of bodyweight

Several methods are available:

- Table of weights (see Table 5.6)
- Calculation
- Weightape
- Weighbridge.

Our 16 hh, three-quarterbred Novice event horse will weigh 500 kg.

### Step two: the horse's appetite

An adult working horse's appetite is about 2.5 per cent of his bodyweight. Foals and lactating broodmares may compensate for their high nutrient requirements by eating more than this.

**Table 5.6**   Approximate bodyweights.

| Height | Bodyweight | |
|---|---|---|
| (hh) | (kg) | (lb) |
| 11 | 120–260 | 264–572 |
| 12 | 230–290 | 506–638 |
| 13 | 290–350 | 638–770 |
| 14 | 350–420 | 770–924 |
| 15 | 420–520 | 924–1144 |
| 16 | 500–600 | 1100–1320 |
| 17 | 600–725 | 1320–1595 |

NB: The values in this table are averages and only approximate.

$$\text{Appetite (kg)} = \frac{\text{bodyweight}}{100} \times 2.5$$

$$\text{Appetite of } 500 \text{ kg horse} = \frac{500}{100} \times 2.5$$
$$= 12.5 \text{ kg } (28 \text{ lb})$$

A 500 kg horse can eat up to 12.5 kg of dry matter per day. Remember that different feeds have different amounts of dry matter in them; a horse will eat much more than 12.5 kg of grass a day because of its high moisture content.

### Step three: calculating the energy for maintenance

The horse requires a minimum amount of energy a day just to stay alive: this is related to the bodyweight of the horse – bigger horses need more feed than smaller ones (see Table 4.3).

$$\text{Energy required for maintenance (MJ DE/day)} = 18 + \frac{\text{bodyweight (kg)}}{10}$$

$$\text{Energy required for a } 500 \text{ kg horse to maintain its bodyweight (MJ DE/day)} = 18 + \frac{500}{10}$$
$$= 18 + 50$$
$$= 68 \text{ MJ DE/day}$$

A 500 kg horse will require 68 MJ DE per day to stay alive and to maintain its bodyweight constant.

## Step four: calculating the energy for work

The amount of energy the horse needs to carry out the work we demand of it depends on the intensity and duration of the work and the horse's bodyweight. The variation in trainer or rider's perception of how much work the horse does has been minimised by giving the work a 'work score' from 1 to 8. Example types of work have been outlined: these are not rigid and you should fit in your horse's individual work load. For each 50 kg of bodyweight, add the following work score (Table 5.7) to calculate the horse's energy requirement for work.

**Table 5.7** Work scoring.

| Type of work | Work score (MJ DE) | Extra energy needed per day by a 500 kg horse (MJ DE/day) |
|---|---|---|
| One hour walking | +1 | 10 |
| One hour walking including some trotting | +2 | 20 |
| One hour including trotting and cantering | +3 | 30 |
| Schooling, dressage and/or jumping | +4 | 40 |
| Novice ODE or hunting one day/week | +5 | 50 |
| Intermediate ODE, hunting 3 days a fortnight, Novice 3-day event | +6 | 60 |
| Advanced ODE, Intermediate 3-day events, hunting 2 days a week | +7 | 70 |
| Racing | +8 | 80 |

A 500 kg Novice one-day event horse will have a score of 5; the extra energy needed to carry out that work will be:

$$\text{work score} \times \frac{\text{bodyweight}}{50}$$

$$= 5 \times \frac{500}{50}$$

$$= 50 \, \text{MJ DE/day}$$

The energy requirement for work is then added to the maintenance requirement to give the total daily energy requirement per day.

Maintenance requirement for 500 kg horse    = 68 MJ DE/day
Work requirement for 500 kg Novice eventer = 50 MJ DE/day
Total energy requirement                = 118 MJ DE/day

### Step five: the forage to concentrate ratio

The horse's work level will determine the amount of energy to come from the forage part of the ration and the amount to come from the concentrate part. Using the revised table of forage to concentrate ratios (Table 5.8) we can calculate how the energy is going to be partitioned.

**Table 5.8**  Forage to concentrate energy partition.

| Work Score | Energy from hay | Energy from concentrates |
|---|---|---|
| Maintenance – Resting | 100 | 0 |
| 1–2 – Light | 75 | 25 |
| 3–5 – Medium | 60 | 40 |
| 6–7 – Hard | 40 | 60 |
| 8 – Fast | 30 | 70 |

Of the total energy requirement (118 MJ DE/day) for our eventer in medium work (work score 5), 60 per cent will come from hay and 40 per cent will come from concentrates.

$$\text{Energy from hay} = \frac{118 \times 60}{100}$$

$$= 71 \, \text{MJ DE}$$

$$\text{Energy from concentrates} = \frac{118 \times 40}{100}$$

$$= 47 \, \text{MJ DE}$$

71MJ DE per day are to be supplied by hay and 47 MJ DE per day by concentrates.

### Step six: making the ration

The next step is to convert these figures into a sensible ration. Using the table of nutrient values (Table 5.9) the energy value of food will be matched with the energy requirements of the feeds.

**Table 5.9**    Nutrient values of common feeds.

|  | Crude protein (%) | Digestible energy (MJ/kg) |
|---|---|---|
| *Hay* | | |
| Average | 4.5–8 | 7–8 |
| Good | 9–10 | 9 |
| Poor | 3.5–6 | 7 |
| *Haylage* | 3.5–6 | 7 |
| *Concentrates* | | |
| Oats | 10 | 11–12 |
| Barley | 9.5 | 13 |
| Maize | 8.5 | 14 |
| Extracted soyabean meal | 44 | 13.3 |
| Peas | 23 | 14 |
| Wheatbran | 15.5 | 11 |
| Sugar beet pulp | 7 | 10.5 |
| Vegetable oil | 0 | 35 |
| *Cubes* | | |
| Horse and Pony | 10 | 9 |
| Performance | 13 | 12 |
| Stud | 15 | 11 |

The 500 kg event horse is to receive 71 MJ DE per day from average quality hay containing 8 MJ DE per kg.

$$\text{Weight of hay to be fed/day} = \frac{71}{8}$$

$$= 9\,\text{kg} \ (20\,\text{lb})$$

The horse is to receive the remaining 47 MJ DE as concentrates. This can be done by feeding a performance horse cube with an energy content of 13 MJ DE/kg.

$$\text{Weight of cubes to be fed/day} = \frac{47}{13}$$

$$= 3.5\,\text{kg} \ (8\,\text{lb})$$

Although perfectly adequate, this is a rather simplistic ration and a mix of feeds is much more likely to be fed (Table 5.10).

Along with his 9 kg (20 lb) of hay our event horse is going to either be fed 3.5 kg (8 lb) of performance cubes or 2 kg oats, 1 kg cubes, 0.5 kg bran and 0.5 kg beet pulp.

The first ration falls within its appetite of 12.5 kg; however the second ration over-faces it by 0.5 kg, because lower energy feeds are being used.

**Table 5.10** The final ration.

| Feed | Quantity (kg) | (lb) | Megajoules provided |
|---|---|---|---|
| Oats | 2 | (4.4) | 24 |
| Sugar beet pulp (dry weight) | 0.5 | (1) | 5 |
| Bran | 0.5 | (1) | 5.5 |
| Performance cubes | 1 | (2.2) | 13 |
| Total | | | 47.5 |

In most cases this small amount may not be of consequence, but a fussy feeder may let you know that the ration is rather too much.

## Step seven: checking the protein level

Energy is the most important aspect of a performance horse's diet, and if good quality feed is being used the protein requirements are likely to be satisfied. However growing youngstock and broodmares will have a high protein requirement and it is important to check the protein level in any ration that you have formulated.

**Table 5.11** Protein requirements of horses.

| Type of activity | Crude protein in the ration (%) |
|---|---|
| Light work | 7.5–8.5 |
| Medium work | 7.5–8.5 |
| Hard work | 9.5–10 |
| Fast work | 9.5–10 |
| Pregnant mare – first 8 months | 7.5–8.5 |
| Pregnant mare – last 3 months | 10 |
| Lactating mare – first 3 months | 12.5 |
| Lactating mare – last 3 months | 11 |
| Stallion | 9.5–10 |
| Weanling | 16 |
| Yearling | 13.5 |
| Two-year-old | 10 |

A horse in medium work requires 7.5–8.5 per cent crude protein. The protein content of the ration can be worked out using the table of nutrient values.

**Table 5.12**   Protein in ration A (hay and cubes).

| Feed | Quantity (kg) | Protein content (%) | Protein in ration (g) |
|------|------|------|------|
| Hay | 9 | 6 | 54 |
| Performance cubes | 3.5 | 13 | 45.5 |
| | 12.5 | | 99.5 |

The percentage of protein in the ration is $\dfrac{99.5}{12.5} = 8$ per cent.

If the hay is low in protein, which is not unusual, and the oat-based ration is used the calculation would look like this:

**Table 5.13**   Protein in ration B (oat-based ration).

| Feed | Quantity (kg) | Protein content (%) | Protein in ration (g) |
|------|------|------|------|
| Hay | 9 | 4.5 | 40.5 |
| Oats | 2 | 10 | 20 |
| Cubes | 1 | 13 | 13 |
| Bran | 0.5 | 15.5 | 7.75 |
| Beet pulp | 0.5 | 7 | 3.5 |
| | 13 | | 84.75 |

The percentage protein in the ration is $84.75/13 = 6.5$ per cent. This is not adequate for a horse in medium work; if the hay is low in protein make sure that the concentrate ration supplies adequate protein by either using a high protein feed like soya, or use a performance cube.

## Step eight: check and adjust the ration

All horses are individuals and must be treated as such. Once a ration has been calculated and is being fed, the horse must be monitored to ensure that the ration is suitable.

- A supply of fresh clean water must be available to the horse at all times.
- The foods must be of good quality and acceptable to the horse – is the horse enjoying its food?

- Not only must the foods satisfy the horse's nutritional requirements, the horse must also be psychologically satisfied; it must not be bored and suffer a craving for roughage.
- The horse's condition must be checked by eye, tape or weighbridge. The horse may be gaining or losing weight. Is this what is wanted? If not alter the ration accordingly. Horses have an optimum performance weight and should be kept as close as possible to this weight.
- The horse's temperament and behaviour may affect the ration fed. Part-bred horses may need more concentrates and less bulk as they are better doers and (usually) more placid. Routine and a quiet yard may save feed as horses are not fretting in their boxes.
- The horse's environment must be monitored; in a cold spell, more food and an extra blanket may be needed. A clipped horse may need more food to maintain its condition if it is not adequately rugged up. In hot weather horses may go off their concentrate ration, because their maintenance requirement has fallen; do not worry unless they start to lose condition.
- Horses must be regularly wormed and have their teeth checked for sharp edges.
- Some horses are poor doers, perhaps due to a gut damaged by worms early in life, and will always need extra attention to their feeding.

## Rations for working horses

Table 5.14 shows the amount of dry food a horse needs to eat every day to maintain condition and bodyweight. A resting horse weighing 500 kg (1100 lb) needs to only eat 7.5 kg (16.5 lb) dry weight of feed per day. As most horses have an appetite of about 2.5% bodyweight (12.5 kg, 27.5 lb per day) it is easy to see why resting horses are prone to put on bodyweight. The same horse in intense work would eat up to 15 kg (33 lb) dry weight of feed daily, in order to fuel the work load.

### Ration for a 16.2 hh (164 cm) dressage horse

- limited period at grass every day
- schooled and/or hacked for 60 mins every day
- two feeds a day

**Table 5.14**  Relationship between bodyweight, work level and appetite.

| Work level and appetite | 200 kg (440 lb) | 400 kg (900 lb) | 450 kg (1000 lb) | 500 kg (1100 lb) | 550 kg (1200 lb) | 600 kg (1320 lb) |
|---|---|---|---|---|---|---|
| *Resting* 1.5% bodyweight | 3 kg (6.5 lb) | 6 kg (13 lb) | 7 kg (15 lb) | 7.5 kg (16.5 lb) | 8 kg (17 lb) | 9 kg (20 lb) |
| *Light work* 2% bodyweight | 4 kg (9 lb) | 8 kg (17 lb) | 9 kg (20 lb) | 10 kg (22 lb) | 11 kg (24 lb) | 12 kg (26.5 lb) |
| *Moderate work* 2.5% bodyweight | 5 kg (11 lb) | 10 kg (22 lb) | 11.5 kg (25 lb) | 12.5 kg (27.5 lb) | 13.5 kg (30 lb) | 14.5 kg (32 lb) |
| *Intense work* 3% bodyweight | 6 kg (13 lb) | 12 kg (26.5 lb) | 13.5 kg (30 lb) | 15 kg (33 lb) | 16.5 kg (36 lb) | 18 kg (40 lb) |

*Step 1: estimation of body weight (Table 5.6)*

$$= 650\,\text{kg}$$

*Step 2: the horse's appetite (Table 5.14)*

$$= 16.25\,\text{kg}\ (36\,\text{lb})$$

*Step 3: energy for maintenance*

$$= 18 + \frac{650}{10}$$
$$= 18 + 65 = 83\,\text{MJ DE/day}$$

*Step 4: energy for work*

$$= 4 \times \frac{650}{50} = 52\,\text{MJ DE}$$

Total energy requirement/day $= 135\,\text{MJ DE}$

*Step 5: forage to concentrate ration*

$$\text{energy from hay} = \frac{135 \times 60}{100} = 81\,\text{MJ DE}$$

$$\text{energy from concentrates} = \frac{135 \times 40}{100} = 54\,\text{MJ DE}$$

*Step 6: making the ration (Table 5.9)*

| Feed | Energy in feed (MJ DE/kg) | Quantity (kg) | (lb) | Energy in ration (MJ DE) |
|------|------|------|------|------|
| Hay | 8 | 10 | 22 | 80 |
| Performance mix | 12 | 2.5 | 5.5 | 30 |
| Sugar beet pulp | 10 | 0.45 | 1 | 4.5 |
| Alfalfa chaff | 10 | 1 | 2.2 | 10 |
| Sunflower oil | 35 | 250 ml | 0.4 pt | 9 |
| Total energy | | | | 133.5 |

*Step 7: checking the protein*

| Feed | Quantity (kg) | (lb) | Protein content (%) | Protein in ration (g) |
|------|------|------|------|------|
| Hay | 10 | 22 | 8 | 80 |
| Performance mix | 2.5 | 5.5 | 12 | 30 |
| Sugar beet pulp | 0.45 | 1 | 7 | 3 |
| Alfalfa chaff | 1 | 2.2 | 15 | 15 |
| Sunflower oil | 250 ml | 0.4 pt | 0 | |
| Total | 14 kg | | | 128 |
| % protein in ration | 9% | | | |

*Step 8: check and adjust the ration*

As the horse is out to grass during the day, the hay ration would be adjusted depending on the quantity and quality of grass available. The horse would be given electrolytes to replace the salts lost in sweat. If cereals are used instead of mix a general purpose supplement would be added to the ration.

## Ration for a 16 hh (159 cm) novice one day event horse

- limited period at grass every day
- schooled and/or hacked for 60–90 minutes every day
- three feeds a day.

*Step 1: estimation of bodyweight (Table 5.6)*

= 500 kg

*Step 2: the horse's appetite (Table 5.14)*

= 12.5 kg (27.5 lb)

*Step 3: energy for maintenance*

$$= 18 + \frac{500}{10}$$

$$= 18 + 50 = 68 \, \text{MJ DE/day}$$

*Step 4: energy for work*

$$= 5 \times \frac{500}{50} = 50 \, \text{MJ DE}$$

Total energy requirement/day $= 118 \, \text{MJ DE}$

*Step 5: forage to concentrate ration*

$$\text{energy from hay} = \frac{118 \times 60}{100} = 71 \, \text{MJ DE}$$

$$\text{energy from concentrates} = \frac{118 \times 40}{100} = 47 \, \text{MJ DE}$$

*Step 6: making the ration (Table 5.9)*

| Feed | Energy in feed (MJ DE/kg) | Quantity (kg) | (lb) | Energy in ration (MJ DE) |
|------|------|------|------|------|
| Hay | 8 | 9 | 20 | 72 |
| Performance mix | 12 | 2.5 | 5.5 | 30 |
| Sugar beet pulp | 10 | 0.45 | 1 | 4.5 |
| Alfalfa chaff | 10 | 0.45 | 1 | 4.5 |
| Sunflower oil | 35 | 250 ml | 0.4 pt | 9 |
| Total energy | | | | 120 |

*Step 7: checking the protein*

| Feed | Quantity (kg) | (lb) | Protein content (%) | Protein in ration (g) |
|------|------|------|------|------|
| Hay | 9 | 20 | 8 | 72 |
| Performance mix | 2.5 | 5.5 | 12 | 30 |
| Sugar beet pulp | 0.45 | 1 | 7 | 3 |
| Alfalfa chaff | 0.45 | 1 | 15 | 7 |
| Sunflower oil | 250 ml | 0.4 pt | 0 | 0 |
| Total | 12.5 kg | | | 112 |
| % protein in ration | 9% | | | |

*Step 8: check and adjust the ration*

As the horse is out to grass during the day, the hay ration would be adjusted depending on the quantity and quality of grass available. The horse would be given electrolytes to replace the salts lost in sweat. If cereals are used instead of mix a general purpose supplement would be added to the ration.

## Ration for a 16 hh (159 cm) advanced three-day event horse

- limited period at grass every day
- schooled and/or hacked for 60–90 minutes every day; fast work every four days
- three feeds a day.

*Step 1: estimation of bodyweight (Table 5.6)*

$$= 500\,\text{kg}$$

*Step 2: the horse's appetite (Table 5.14)*

$$= 12.5\,\text{kg} \ (27.5\,\text{lb})$$

*Step 3: energy for maintenance*

$$= 18 + \frac{500}{10}$$

$$= 18 + 50 = 68\,\text{MJ DE/day}$$

*Step 4: energy for work*

$$= 7 \times \frac{500}{50} = 70\,\text{MJ DE}$$

Total energy requirement/day $= 138\,\text{MJ DE}$

*Step 5: forage to concentrate ration*

$$\text{energy from hay} = \frac{138 \times 40}{100} = 55\,\text{MJ DE}$$

$$\text{energy from concentrates} = \frac{138 \times 60}{100} = 83\,\text{MJ DE}$$

*Step 6: making the ration (Table 5.9)*

| Feed | Energy in feed (MJ DE/kg) | Quantity (kg) | (lb) | Energy in ration (MJ DE) |
|---|---|---|---|---|
| Hay | 8 | 6.5 | 14 | 52 |
| Performance mix | 12 | 5.5 | 12 | 66 |
| Sugar beet pulp | 10 | 0.45 | 1 | 4.5 |
| Alfalfa chaff | 10 | 0.45 | 1 | 4.5 |
| Sunflower oil | 35 | 250 ml | 0.4 pt | 9 |
| Total energy | | | | 136 |

*Step 7: checking the protein*

| Feed | Quantity (kg) | (lb) | Protein content (%) | Protein in ration (g) |
|---|---|---|---|---|
| Hay | 6.5 | 14 | 8 | 52 |
| Performance mix | 5.5 | 12 | 12 | 66 |
| Sugar beet pulp | 0.45 | 1 | 7 | 3 |
| Alfalfa chaff | 9.45 | 1 | 15 | 7 |
| Sunflower oil | 250 ml | 0.4 pt | 0 | 0 |
| Total | 13 | | | 128 |
| % protein in ration | 9.8 | | | |

*Step 8: check and adjust the ration*

As the horse is out to grass during the day, the hay ration would be adjusted depending on the quantity and quality of grass available. Feeding haylage or better quality hay would reduce the bulk of the ration and increase both energy and protein if required. The horse would be given electrolytes to replace the salts lost in sweat. If cereals are used instead of mix a general purpose supplement would be added to the ration.

Horses will vary in their reaction to and acceptance of a ration. The ration can be altered to cater for the horse which tends to go off its feed by reducing the bulk and increasing the concentrates so that the total weight of the ration is reduced but the energy content stays the same (see Table 15.5). Conversely for the horse that always appears to be hungry, the bulk can be increased and the concentrates reduced so that the total weight of the ration is increased; but, again, the energy content stays the same.

**Table 5.15**  Adjusting the ration to cater for individual horses.

| Adjustment to concentrate | Concentrate (kg) | (lb) | Adjustment to hay | Hay (kg) | (lb) | Total (kg) | (lb) |
|---|---|---|---|---|---|---|---|
| Original ration | 5 | 11 | – | 7.5 | 16.5 | 12.5 | 27.5 |
| *Poor appetite* | | | | | | | |
| Increase by 5% | 5.25 | 11.5 | Decrease by 10% | 6.75 | 15 | 12 | 26.5 |
| or | | | or | | | | |
| Increase by 10% | 5.5 | 12 | Decrease by 20% | 6 | 13 | 11.5 | 25 |
| *Hungry horse* | | | | | | | |
| Decrease by 5% | 4.75 | 10.5 | Increase by 10% | 8.25 | 18 | 13 | 28.5 |
| or | | | or | | | | |
| Decrease by 10% | 4.5 | 10 | Increase by 20% | 9 | 20 | 13.5 | 30 |

# Chapter 6
# Grassland Management

Detailed and authoritative texts have been written about grassland management, but there is still a lack of understanding among horse owners about the day-to-day care of their horses' paddocks. Too often we still see horses grazing horse-sick, ragwort infested paddocks. You clean your tack and scrub out the feedroom, so why not care for your pasture in the same way?

Many owners of competition horses regard the paddock as just somewhere for the horse to stretch its legs and have a roll, taking no account of the nutritional value of the grass at all. Other horses have to rely on the grass for all their nutritional needs in the summer, as they are out 24 hours a day. Good grassland management is time-consuming and requires a certain amount of capital outlay. One of the major problems is that the horse owner is not always the paddock owner, and is not in a position to initiate new management routines. The following chapter outlines some important principles of grassland management and then puts these together as a grassland year for easy reference.

## Drainage

Ideally any paddock used for horses would be reasonably well drained. Good drainage allows air to enter the soil so that roots and soil organisms can develop and improve the soil structure. Well-drained soil warms up sooner in the spring, giving earlier grass, and also makes the soil firmer so that horses can stay out longer in the autumn. Plants in well-drained soil develop better root systems so that they are more resistant to drought.

If the drainage is poor any money spent on upgrading pasture is largely wasted, yet correcting a drainage problem is very expensive. If your horses are grazing an established pasture there are several routine jobs that can help maintain the drainage system:

- Keep ditches clear – they may be all that is needed to drain a field.

Ditches should be fenced off so that horses cannot damage the sides of the ditch and cannot fall in.

- Keep culverts in good condition (culverts are the pipes which take a ditch under gate openings).
- Keep the junction between the ditch and the piped mains clear; there may be a silt trap which gets blocked up.

## Desirable grass varieties

Grass does not just grow of its own accord. To maintain high quality permanent pasture, farmers have to treat the grass as a cultivated crop, including grazing. Modern agriculture has seen an increase in highly-fertilised permanent pastures and leys, which are grasses planted with the intention of ploughing them up within a few years. These swards tend to have an open texture, which poaches easily, and tend to be stony due to ploughing, while old pastures have a thick cushion of grass that is better for horses. These highly-fertilised permanent pastures and leys are often too lush for resting horses, barren broodmares, pregnant mares and youngstock and can lead to laminitis, obesity and growth problems. This means that there is a large degree of skill in creating and maintaining a pasture that will provide useful, nutritious grazing and be suitable for horses.

The grasses used in horse paddocks should have the following characteristics:

- palatability
- persistence – the ability to withstand hard grazing and cutting
- winter hardiness
- resistance to disease
- varying heading (flowering) dates, to ensure an even spread of growth
- moderate yield – too high a yield may cause digestive upsets
- moderate digestibility – too much or too little fibre in the grass is not desirable for horses.

A basic horse paddock grass seed mixture will contain

- two perennial ryegrasses (*Lolium perenne*): 50 per cent
- two creeping red fescues (*Festuca rubra*): 25 per cent
- crested dog's tail (*Cynosurus cristatus*): 5–10 per cent
- rough or smooth stalked meadow grass: 5–10 per cent
- wild white clover: 1–2 per cent.

Some timothy (Fig. 6.1) or cocksfoot may also be used. Seeding rates vary from 10–18 kg per acre (25–45 kg per ha) depending on the detailed make up of the mixture. These grass species have been chosen for certain characteristics:

**perennial ryegrass** is very versatile and does well under all types of soil and is very persistent in good rich soil.

**creeping red fescue** is palatable and has good nutritional quality, it thrives under difficult conditions, and is often used for sports turf.

**crested dog's tail** is very palatable to horses.

**smooth stalked meadow grass** (*Poa pratensis*), also known as Kentucky blue grass, is ideal for light sandy soils as it is able to withstand drought.

**rough stalked meadow grass** (*Poa trivialis*) is palatable and likes moist, rich soils; it gives a good 'bottom' to a sward.

**wild white clover** (*Trifolium repens*) is a nitrogen-producing legume, which can enhance soil fertility and is able to withstand drought. Excessive amounts of clover should be avoided.

Herbs may be included in the mixture or may be planted in a separate strip. Acceptable pasture herbs include dandelion, narrow-leaved plantain, chicory, yarrow, burnet, sheep's parsley and wild garlic.

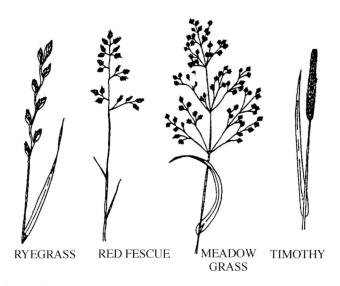

RYEGRASS    RED FESCUE    MEADOW    TIMOTHY
                          GRASS

**Fig. 6.1**  Types of grasses.

# Weed control

Apart from the possibility that they may be poisonous, weeds compete with grasses for space, light, water and soil nutrients. They reduce the quality and quantity of grass available for grazing. The most common weeds to affect paddocks include

- nettles
- docks
- creeping thistle
- spear thistle
- chickweed

- buttercup
- ragwort
- rush horsetails
- foxglove.

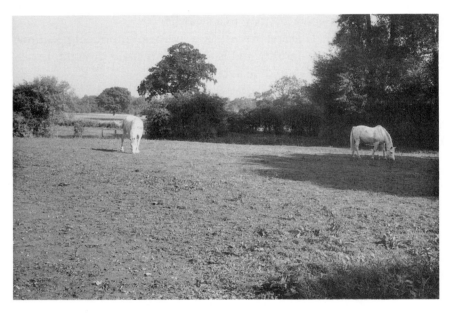

**Fig. 6.2**   A well-kept, weed-free pony paddock.

The Injurious Weeds Order permits the serving on the occupier of any land of a notice requiring them to cut or destroy specified weeds; if they fail to comply they are liable to be fined. Injurious weeds include spear thistle, creeping thistle, curled dock, broad leaved dock and ragwort.

## Methods of control

Methods of control fall into two main areas, physical control and chemical control.

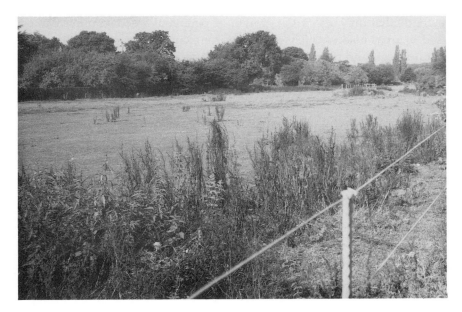

**Fig. 6.3**   A weed-infested, overgrazed paddock.

*Physical control*

Mowing or topping is generally done using a tractor mounted mower, and should be carried out about five times during the growing season to be effective. Once cut, the weeds must be removed from the paddock or they will drop their seeds. Also some poisonous weeds such as ragwort are more palatable when dead. Mowing encourages the grass to grow at a uniform height and leaves no areas of long grass, improving the appearance of the grazing. It also encourages the grass to grow by tillering and producing more leaf, which is the most nutritious part of the plant. Any clover in the sward will be too short to be affected by mowing. Machinery should only be used by a person over 13 years of age.

Pulling by hand is only effective for certain types of weed, and is not practical for large areas. Pulling needs to be done several times a year and must be carried out before flowering and seeding. Care must be taken not to leave any part of the root in the ground, as this will allow the weed to regrow.

*Chemical control*

Spraying from a tractor is a quick and effective method of weed control. Sprays actually kill the weed and can prove more economical than other methods that only check the growth of perennial weeds. Sprays can be used in areas inaccessible to a mower, for example along fence lines and around trees, and they are also effective against low growing weeds that cannot be cut by a mower. Take care that the spray does not kill the clover.

Spraying should be carried out twice a year, and it is necessary to make alternative arrangements for grazing for the 14 days after spraying, while the weeds die back and are collected and burnt. Weather conditions can cause variation in the results and the reaction of the plants to spraying.

Spot spraying is selective and is carried out by a person with a knapsack sprayer. It can be useful for small areas or clumps of weeds, and as you are being selective it is not going to harm the clover all over the field. As with tractor spraying it is necessary to remove the dead weeds from the field, and to remove the stock for up to 14 days after spraying.

Take care to read the directions for spraying and follow the guidelines given by the manufacturer of the weedkiller you choose.

## Fencing

Safety is the major consideration when selecting fencing, and its suitability for the horses in question. It must be stock proof, unlikely to inflict injury, high enough at the top and low enough at the bottom, and it should discourage horses from leaning on it or chewing it. Types of fencing include:

- post and rail
- wire mesh
- plain wire
- electric fencing.

The final choice will depend on cost and appearance but it is always preferable to get the best that you can afford; anything else is false economy.

## Acreage of grassland required per horse

The area of grassland required per horse will vary depending on several factors:

- type of horse/pony
- supplementary food available

- time of year
- soil type
- the pasture management capability of the horse owner.

A small pony can be kept on 0.5–1 acres (0.2–0.4 ha), providing that the droppings are picked up, the paddock is fertilised and kept weed-free. In general the ideal is 1.5–4 acres (0.6–1.6 ha) per pony/horse divided into three or four; this will allow one paddock to be rested at any one time. Two and a half acres (1 ha) of fertile, well managed grassland (for example in the stud situation) will support 3–4 horses or 4–6 ponies. Average grassland will maintain one horse per acre (0.4 ha) all year round or two horses for the summer only. Typical badly-managed paddocks will only support one horse for every 2.5 acres (1 ha).

# The grassland year

## To start with

One of the first principles of good management of a small area of grassland is to divide the field so that one part may be rested, sprayed or fertilised. It is probably worthwhile to have a soil analysis carried out. Make sure that the company know that the field is for grazing horses. The analysis will tell you whether you need to lime the field and how much nitrogen (N), phosphate (P) and potash (K) are needed. You can then follow this guide to the events of the grassland year.

# Winter

Turning out horses in winter can damage the sward extensively. The wetter the soil and the more horses on the paddock, the greater the damage. The horses' hooves cut through the sward and disrupt the soil structure and the ground is said to be poached. The hooves destroy leaves, growing points and roots of the grass and spread mud on the grass, making it unpalatable.

Winter grazing is reduced in both quantity and quality. Horses and ponies living out will require additional feeding even if the field looks well covered. Once the horses have grazed the available grass it will not be replaced by natural regrowth; long-lasting damage may be caused by a reduction in the density of the grass plants, allowing more poaching to take place. This damage can be reduced by management of the following factors:

- grazing management
- soil conditions
- quality of the sward.

## Grazing management

The only way to protect the grassland completely is to remove all stock before the land gets too wet. However the number of horses on the land in the summer will affect the density and resilience of the sward; over-grazed pasture poaches more rapidly than well preserved grassland. Fewer horses all year round will help keep the grassland in good shape.

Alternatively one paddock can be 'sacrificed' while the others are rested. In the spring this paddock will require extensive renovation but the others will be available for grazing or conservation. The newly-renovated paddock should be rested through the following winter.

## Soil conditions

The type of soil will affect the amount of water that it holds – sandy soils are free-draining and poach less easily than heavy, readily-saturated clay soils. It makes sense to have a well drained paddock on good soil for winter use, ideally, a field sloping gently towards a suitable outlet, such as a ditch, pond or stream that is fenced off from the horses. The field should have well maintained ditches; the proper maintenance of the ditches incorporated into the field drainage system can greatly reduce the water held in the soil, in turn reducing poaching and damage to the grassland. Major drainage is an expensive undertaking and an alternative is mole draining. A large round ball is sunk into the soil and pulled along; this creates a channel under the ground, allowing water to flow away. On the surface only a small slit is visible.

## Quality of the sward

Recently-seeded grassland is more susceptible to damage than old pasture. Old well-established turf is the best; grasses that form a thick springy mat can help to prevent horse's hooves penetrating into the soil. These grasses are the varieties most common on hill pasture. They do not offer high nutritional value but the feeding value of any grass in the winter is minimal. Whatever grasses there are in the sward, a field that has been heavily grazed in the summer and left with little grass cover will not fare well if grazed in winter.

## Other points

Fencing and gateways come under more pressure during winter than in summer. Hungry stock may chew rails, eat hedges and chew the bark from trees. Make sure that the fencing is sturdy with no gaps for a hungry horse to squeeze through.

Gates are a bottleneck, getting twice as much treading as other areas. Siting a gate at the top of a hill can reduce the water that collects around it. Putting down sand or gravel will help water to drain quickly and will raise the ground level up above that of the water. The same can be done around water troughs. A field with good hedges and a few trees will provide some natural shelter for the horses. Be careful that there are no poisonous trees or plants within reach and protect the trees from being eaten.

When choosing a field for winter grazing remember:

- Use a well drained field on free-draining soil.
- A gently-sloping field will aid drainage.
- Choose a well established sward, preferably permanent pasture, with thick springy turf and good grass cover.
- Take extra care over vulnerable areas such as gateways.
- Check fences and hedges for weak spots that may let horses escape.
- Reduce the stocking density to a minimum.

## Getting grassland ready for spring

As the weeks go by and the days become longer horse owners begin to think about turning out their grass-hungry horses. However, the pasture they left in the autumn will need some help if it is to provide good quality spring grass – so what can be done to prepare horse paddocks for spring grazing?

### Harrowing

Assuming that the pasture is in good heart and not suffering from poor drainage, the first step is to harrow. Harrowing involves a tractor dragging linked chains with spikes attached over the grass; this will remove dead and matted grass that is clogging-up the base of the plants. This dead material prevents air from reaching the plant roots and the soil.

Poorly aerated soil and roots do not help grass growth; this is why lawns are regularly spiked. The dead grass is unavoidable and may come from frost damaged grass dying back and settling at the base of the plants. Harrowing will also help spread any mole-hills or piles of droppings that may still be in the field; it can also aid in the levelling of poached or cut-up areas by breaking up the rough soil surface.

Paddocks should be harrowed regularly during the spring to ensure that droppings are broken up and spread out. If the paddock is small enough, the droppings can be collected by hand. This is tedious and time-consuming but also a very effective way of keeping the grass palatable and as parasite-free as possible. Take care not to over-harrow with a tined or spiked harrow as this may rip the grass plants out of the soil or weaken the roots so that they are pulled up by grazing animals or scorched by the sun.

## Soil nutrient testing

Soil nutrient testing should be carried out every three years. Most British grassland is naturally acid, often below pH 5.5, while the optimum pH for grass growth is 6.0–6.5. A higher pH results in more vigorous grass growth and improved mineral content, particularly calcium and phosphorus. Well-managed grassland contains a calcium to phosphorus ratio of 2:1 – ideal for the growing horse. Ground limestone, chalk or another calcium-containing substance needs to be added every few years to counteract the natural acidifying effect of rain. A soil test should recommend how much lime to apply.

Phosphorus and potassium are also needed in considerable quantities by the grass; the level of these nutrients in the soil is expressed as an index, and the aim should be to maintain grassland at index 2.

**Table 6.1**  Fertiliser input needed to achieve a soil index of 2 (kg/ha).

| Soil index | 0 | 1 | 2 | 2+ |
|---|---|---|---|---|
| Phosphorus (P205) | 60+ | 40 | 20 | 0 |
| Potash (K20) | 60 | 30 | 0 | 0 |

These levels should be reduced if organic manure is also applied.

## Fertilising

After harrowing has taken place the next step is to fertilise the field. Assuming that there are no severe deficiencies in any particular soil nutrient, a top dressing of nitrogen can be applied. Many horse owners are worried about using nitrogen because they associate it with rich dairy cow pastures which can cause problems like laminitis and epiphysitis in horses. However nitrogen is necessary because it is vital to the healthy growth of all plants and is easily leached or washed out of the soil during the winter. The most common way for nitrogen to be applied is as 'bag muck', that is, an artificially produced granular form. Nowadays it is possible to buy slow-release organic fertilisers which are ideal for horse paddocks that require slow, steady grass growth. Clover in the pasture can replace nitrogen naturally by bacteria living in the clover roots fixing atmospheric nitrogen. If the grazing is not to be used until later in the year and there is adequate clover, artificial nitrogen may not be needed at all.

If you regularly spread the droppings potash may not be necessary, but if the droppings are removed, or a hay crop taken, a low level of potash may be needed. Phosphate may well be needed every two to three years and a liming material applied every three to seven years to bring the pH to around 6.5. Regular soil sampling will help you decide which fertilisers to use and how much of each nutrient. Intensively-run horse enterprises may need to fertilise throughout the year, while spring and autumn application is adequate for most privately owned paddocks.

Once the field has been fertilised it must not be grazed until the fertiliser has dissolved into the ground. This gives you the chance to do any weed control that may be necessary. Some organic fertilisers may be safe enough for horses to graze fields that have been recently dressed.

## Rolling

The paddock should be rolled either before or after fertilising. If a heavy roller is used after top-dressing the field it helps to incorporate the nitrogen granules into the ground. Rolling consolidates the soil and helps to flatten out areas damaged by poaching; loose stones are pushed into the soil so that they are less likely to be flicked up by a mower or other implement that may be used later in the year, and rolling encourages the grass to tiller and so form more leaf. This happens because the growing shoots are gently crushed and secondary growth points take over. More leaves are produced, and combined with the recent application of nitrogen this causes more grass growth earlier in the year.

When should these jobs be done? To begin early in the year risks nitrogen being leached out of the soil before the plants become active. To begin late wastes important growing time. Different methods have been used over the years to pinpoint the time to start treating pastures. One is the 'T-sum', which involves adding up all the average daily temperatures from 1 January each year; when the total reaches 200 it is time to fertilise your fields. However this method does not allow for sub-zero temperatures or for regional variations. In some years the T-sum may be reached as early as February, while in other years it may not be reached until April. Another method uses soil temperature as a guide: once a temperature of 5.5°C is reached at a depth of 10 cm (4 in) the initial application of fertiliser is made. This is usually about mid-March, but the field should be fertilised by the beginning of April even if the soil temperature is still low.

Preparing paddocks too early can be a waste of time and money and can seriously damage wet land; leaving it too late risks missing out on early grass growth and thus shortening the growing season. As a guide, if the land is dry enough to get a tractor on it without damage, the preparations for spring should begin during March, but in any case should not be left any later than the beginning of April.

## Summer grassland management

During the summer fields should be harrowed weekly if the droppings are not being picked up, preferably during warm, drying weather to desiccate the worm larvae. Even if droppings are collected harrowing should take place once a month. Horses are fussy grazers and often leave rank areas around their droppings. The sward should be 'topped' regularly to a length of 10–15 cm (4–6 in); this prevents these areas seeding and poor quality grass species taking over.

Depending on the weather there may be large quantities of grass, allowing you to shut up a paddock for hay making. The remaining paddocks should be grazed on a rotational basis, giving adequate time to rest and recover before putting horses back on. If cattle are kept they can 'mop up' the rougher grasses once the horses are removed; this also helps break the worm cycle.

Any weeds remaining after the spring spraying should be pulled up and removed before they go to seed.

## Autumn grassland management

Pasture quality declines rapidly in the autumn. Even if there appears to be a large quantity of herbage, watch for horses losing weight and be ready to supplement their diet. Farmyard manure is usually spread in the autumn, and applying lime may be more convenient in the autumn, if horses are going to be taken off for the winter.

## Grassland management of the worm problem

What a relief it is to turn our horses out into the field in the spring for a good dose of 'Dr Green'. Back to their natural life style of grazing and continually moving around in search of the best forage – but is this so healthy? Along with the fresh spring grass the horses also take in mouthfuls of parasitic worm larvae. In the wild the horse roams over large areas of grassland, grazing and constantly moving forwards – leaving its droppings behind. Keeping horses in confined paddocks with high stocking rates is not natural; the horse is forced to graze close to dung containing larvae and is always being re-infected, resulting in a high parasite burden.

Environmental and management factors can directly influence the development and survival of the parasite population on the grass, and combined with an efficient worming programme, can greatly reduce the threat of harmful parasite infestation.

Parasitic worms have complex life cycles, with larvae or eggs passing into the horse's gut, migrating and developing into egg-laying adults. The eggs or larvae leave the horse and return to the pasture to start the cycle over again as the horse eats the contaminated grass.

## 'Clean' pasture

One way of reducing the worm burden is to start with 'clean' pasture – this is especially important when larval populations are high in the spring, summer and autumn. Large numbers of larvae on the grass coincide with optimal conditions for grass growth and horses tend to get maximum exposure when there is an abundance of good grazing. Land that has not been grazed by horses since the previous autumn and which is then used for hay or silage is the 'cleanest'. If the grass has been grazed in the spring, then used for conservation and subsequently grazed by sheep or cattle, it too will be 'clean' for horses to use the following spring.

## Rotational grazing

A three year rotation of grazing can provide an efficient method of reducing worm infestation on the pasture, and so provide cleaner grazing. It is important to start the grazing season with horses that have been regularly wormed through the winter and ideally to use a paddock that has not been grazed by horses the previous year. The land is divided into thirds, one of which is grown for hay or silage, while the other two are grazed by horses and sheep or cattle. The following year a different third is used for conservation and this rotation continues as shown in Fig. 6.4.

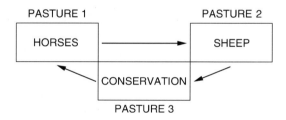

**Fig. 6.4**   Rotational grazing.

## 'Leader-follower' system

You must also consider the vulnerability of different horses – young foals are open targets for infection, especially by ascarids, which multiply rapidly in horses up to nine months of age and quickly contaminate the pasture. Fortunately the young horse's resistance increases with age, reducing the number of egg-laying adults and the consequent pasture contamination. However the eggs are long-lived and can survive from one year to the next, which means that foals should not be grazed on the same paddock year after year. A 'leader-follower' system of grazing can be adopted (Fig. 6.5), where the susceptible youngsters are grazed on the cleanest pasture followed by the more resistant adult horses. However clean pasture must be used at the beginning of the season.

| FIELD | 1 | 2 | 3 | 4 |
|---|---|---|---|---|
| PERIOD 1 | MARES AND FOALS | CONSERVATION | YOUNG HORSES | OLDER HORSES |
| 2 | OLDER HORSES | MARES AND FOALS | CONSERVATION | YOUNG HORSES |
| 3 | YOUNG HORSES | OLDER HORSES | MARES AND FOALS | CONSERVATION |

**Fig. 6.5**  Leader-follower system.

## Zero grazing

Even using rotational grazing and a 'leader-follower' system, as the horses graze they will be re-infecting themselves, and this three-year rotation will only help reduce the burden, not remove it altogether. Success will also depend on the number of horses grazing the paddocks – if the stocking rate is high the worm infestation will also be higher. There is one system that can reduce the worm burden dramatically: zero grazing. The grass is cut in the field and carried to the horses so that it is never contaminated by droppings. This is all very well for the dairy farmer but quite beyond most of us.

## Removal of dung

At this point you are probably thinking that you have no hope of controlling your horses' worm infestation by grazing management because you simply do not have the land or the equipment. Don't give up: there are other methods that you can use on a smaller grazing area.

Most larvae and eggs are passed onto pasture via the droppings, so that it makes sense to reduce infestation by picking up the droppings twice a week. The method used will depend on the size of paddock being cleared; a wheelbarrow and fork are adequate for small areas but a vacuum machine is more practical for larger areas. Removing the droppings also reduces tainted areas that the horse will not graze.

Removing the dung is most important when the weather is warm (10–35°C) and damp as these are ideal conditions for rapid larval development. At temperatures above 35°C larvae develop but do not survive long, but eggs can be very resistant and stay dormant until conditions are better for them.

## Harrowing

Harrowing fields in hot, dry weather to spread the droppings so that they dry out is an effective way of reducing larvae on the pasture, but will not affect the eggs to any great extent. Horses should not graze the newly-harrowed field until the dung has dried out and larvae cannot be picked up. Some schools of thought believe that harrowing sours the whole field, making the grass less palatable, and spreading eggs and larvae over the whole area so that if the weather changes and it rains it could make matters worse. Much depends on the stocking rate; if there are large numbers of horses, collecting the droppings is preferable.

## Worming

It is important to worm any new horses before turning them out with established horses; one heavily-infected horse can dramatically increase the threat to the others.

Controlling parasites by grassland management can only be effective if a regular, efficient worming programme is used on all horses throughout the year. If worming is used in conjunction with one or more of the methods outlined here it is possible to reduce the worm burden on the pasture and hence in the horse itself.

## Toxic weeds

There are many plants and trees that are poisonous to horses. Sometimes the horse may avoid eating the fresh weed, but it may become palatable when cut and wilted, or in hay. The danger is always greater when hungry horses are kept in weed-infested horse-sick paddocks.

The toxicity of any plant will vary in different parts of the plant and will be affected by the time of year, stage of growth, climate and soil conditions. Horses will also vary in their susceptibility to different plants, depending on their age, condition, management, state of health, worm burden, and the type and quantity of other forage eaten at the same time as the poisonous plant. An individual horse's metabolism will determine how quickly the toxin is excreted in the urine, and thus how resistant the horse is to the plant.

Some poisons have a cumulative effect as the horse grazes small amounts of the plant. Gradually the horse's temperament, disease resistance and condition are affected as the toxins build up, finally producing clinical signs of ill-health. Weeds like ragwort, bracken and horsetails have a cumulative effect. Other poisons are very toxic and small amounts of the plant can kill a horse very quickly: yew falls into this category.

Plants found in the UK that are poisonous to horses in fresh and dried form include: horsetails, bracken, yew, hellebores, columbines, monkshood, larkspurs, poppies, greater celandine, St John's wort, corncockle, soapwort, sandwort, chickweed, flax, buckthorn, alder buckthorn, lupins, laburnum, cowbane, hemlock, water dropwort, white bryony, hemp, rhododendron, sowbread, pimpernels, thornapple, henbane, deadly nightshade, black nightshade, potato, foxglove, ragwort, lily of the valley, fritillary, meadow saffron, herb paris, irises, black bryony and darnel.

## *The effects of common poisonous plants*

### *Ragwort*

Ragwort (Fig. 6.6) is one of the most common causes of poisoning in horses in the UK. At the end of July and beginning of August many poorly managed, over-grazed horse paddocks will be infested with this bright yellow weed. Ragwort contains an alkaloid that causes permanent liver damage, called seneciosis. Horses with a ragwort-damaged liver need a balanced diet with good quality protein, supplemented with B vitamins and trace elements. Groundsel also contains the same poison as ragwort, but at lower levels.

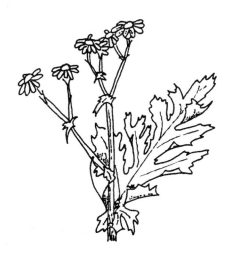

**Fig. 6.6**   Ragwort.

Ragwort is not usually grazed fresh, but it is palatable when cut and wilted, either in hay or by the horse's hooves in the paddock. The effect is cumulative and signs may develop months after the first exposure to the weed. The horse loses weight and is depressed, and may wander aimlessly in advanced cases. Hay containing 15 per cent ragwort will kill a horse over a period of time, but up to 5 kg must be eaten before a horse will show signs of ragwort poisoning. There may be many horses suffering from sub-clinical or low-level ragwort poisoning, leading to loss of condition and susceptibility to other problems, such as laminitis.

### Yew

Yew (Fig. 6.7) is the most toxic plant in the UK. Little more than 100 g or one mouthful of it will cause sudden cardiac arrest and rapid death in the horse. Yew is not usually eaten but may be attractive to the horse if there is snow on the ground or grazing is very scarce. Even dead leaves below a tree are dangerous; take care that hedge clippings are not dumped over the hedge into the horse's field. There is no known antidote.

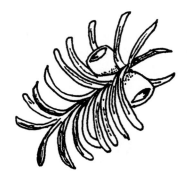

**Fig. 6.7**   Yew, showing leaves and berries.

### Laburnum

Laburnum is the second most poisonous plant in the UK. It is one of the family of legumes that also includes broom and lupins. Laburnum seeds are highly toxic, containing alkaloids that can kill within a few hours of the horse ingesting as little as 500 g. Laburnum is frequently found as a decorative tree in urban hedgerows and garden boundaries – beware of overhanging branches which the horse may reach or which may drop seeds into the paddock.

*Bracken*

Bracken is another serious cause of losses of stock. Although it is usually avoided it is so abundant on marginal and hill land that hungry horses will eat it when other food is scarce. Horses must usually eat bracken for 30–60 days before signs of poisoning are seen but these can appear even if none has been eaten for two to three weeks. Horses lose weight, become weak and eventually become uncoordinated. The toxin is thiaminase, which breaks down thiamine (vitamin $B_1$). Horses can make a full recovery if the condition is treated quickly: treatment consists of daily doses of thiamine hydrochloride to restore body levels. Horses should be removed from the bracken-infested pasture.

*Horsetail*

Horsetail or marestail is found in wetter and colder areas than bracken, but the toxin is the same and the signs of poisoning are virtually the same as bracken poisoning. It is rarely eaten fresh but can be dangerous in hay.

## Trace element status

The trace element content of soil, and hence the grass grown in that soil, varies significantly. This will affect the health of the grass and of the horse eating that grass. In the past, when land was used less intensively and organic fertilisers were used, trace element problems were rare and sub-clinical deficiencies less common. However the trace element status of soils can vary widely quite naturally, with clay soils tending to have the highest levels. Drainage of waterlogged soil tends to increase the availability of selenium and zinc but may reduce the availability of iron, manganese, cobalt and molybdenum. Excessive use of nitrogen fertilisers may decrease the concentration of several trace elements but the inter-relationships are very complex. If you are in doubt about the trace element status of the soil and the grass growing on it both soil and plant tissue should be analysed.

Individual trace elements may be deficient or even present in toxic amounts in different regions: for example the poorly-drained soils found in parts of Somerset and Eire may lead to copper deficiency. Soils subject to high rainfall, waterlogging and with a low soil pH tend to produce selenium-deficient pasture; this occurs in areas of the Welsh Hills, Shropshire, north Cornwall and the Scottish borders. Selenium deficiency also occurs on sands and gravels in, for example, Newmarket. Some areas of the USA and Eire may have toxic levels of selenium in the soil. The nutrients most likely to be deficient on the Cotswolds and Chalk Downlands are magnesium, copper and iodine. Alkaline soils tend to lock up manganese and copper so that plant levels may bear little resemblance to soil levels.

Applying minerals to the soil to correct trace element deficiencies is not satisfactory; for some elements the uptake is scant and repeated treatment is needed. Spraying is expensive and supplementary feeding with a suitable source of trace elements is the most practical solution at present.

# Chapter 7
# Diet-related Disorders

This chapter is not intended as a veterinary text. The aim is to help prevent these types of problem from arising by correct feeding practice. To accomplish this it is helpful to understand how these conditions occur and what happens to the horse's body when it is affected by one of these problems.

## Choke

Choke is a term used to describe partial or complete blockage of the gullet or oesophagus. The blockage may be caused by the horse bolting his feed so that it is not properly chewed and moistened; he may be plain greedy, or have a tooth problem making it painful for him to chew.

A horse with choke appears distressed and anxious; he may make repeated movements of the head and neck, arching the neck and then drawing the chin back to the chest or extending the head down to the ground. The horse usually drools and a mixture of food and saliva may run from his nose. This can be very distressing, and if the choke does not spontaneously clear within 30 minutes then veterinary help should be sought. The vet may inject smooth muscle relaxants to help relieve spasms of the oesophagus, after which the choke should clear as the obstruction is allowed to move.

Horses that are prone to choke should be fed well damped feeds; their speed of eating can be slowed down by putting a salt lick or several large stones in the manger. Dry coarse hay should be avoided, and the teeth regularly checked for sharp edges and rasped when necessary.

## Internal parasites

The horse is host to a large variety of internal parasites, most of which are the larval and adult stages of gastrointestinal 'worms'. The most common are shown in Table 7.1.

**Table 7.1**  The major internal parasites of horses.

| Type | Species | Development site Adults | Larvae |
|------|---------|-------------------------|--------|
| *Large strongyles:* | | | |
| (redworm) | *Strongylus vulgaris* | Caecum | Intestinal arteries |
| | *S. edentatus* | Colon | Liver |
| | *Triodontophorus spp.* | Caecum/colon | Intestinal wall |
| *Small strongyles* | *Trichonema spp.* | Caecum/colon | Intestinal wall |
| *Ascarids:* | | | |
| (roundworms) | *Parascaris equorum* | Small intestine | Liver/lungs |
| Bot | *Gasterophilus spp.* | Bot flies | Stomach |
| Threadworms | *Strongyloides westeri* | Small intestine | Various tissues |
| Pinworms | *Oxyuris equi* | Colon/rectum | Intestinal wall |
| Lungworm | *Dictyocaulus arnfieldi* | Bronchi of lungs | Lymphatics and lungs |
| Tapeworms | *Anoplocephala perfoliata* | Ileum/caecum | (Intermediate host) |

Horses are susceptible to different types of worm at different stages in their life (see Table 7.2). Of primary importance in the young foal are ascarids and threadworms, while the redworms (*Strongylus vulgaris, Strongylus endentatus* and *Trichonema species*) are by far the most serious worm infections in older horses and can ultimately cause death.

**Table 7.2**  Types of worm affecting horses at different ages.

| Foal | Up to 3 years | Adult |
|------|---------------|-------|
| Threadworm | Large roundworm | Redworm |
| Large roundworm or | Redworm | Small strongyles |
| white worm | Small strongyles | Bots |
| | Bots | Tapeworm |
| | Tapeworm | Lungworm |
| | Lungworm | Pinworm |
| | Pinworm | |

Worm control is a vital aspect of any horse management programme, and can be made more effective by an understanding of the life-cycles of these parasites and a knowledge of the drugs available for their control.

## *Ascarids (Parascaris equorum)*

These large worms may be 30 cm (12 inches) long and as thick as a pencil (Fig. 7.1). An adult egg-laying female living in the small intestine can lay

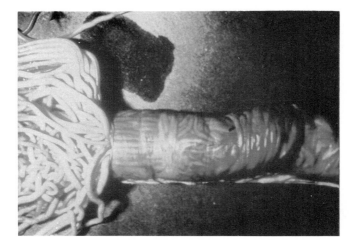

**Fig. 7.1**   Ascarids *(Parascaris equorum)* in small intestine.

200 000 to 1 million eggs per day. The eggs have a tough, sticky outer coat which makes them very resistant to disinfectants and the environment, allowing them to survive for up to three years outside the horse (Fig. 7.2). Infective larvae develop inside the egg; when eaten by the foal, they hatch in the foal's gut and burrow through the gut wall, migrating via the blood stream to the liver and lungs (Fig. 7.3). The larvae are coughed up, swallowed and undergo their final development to become egg-laying adults inside the small intestine. It takes 8–12 weeks from infection (the foal eating the eggs) for the larvae to mature and for eggs to start being

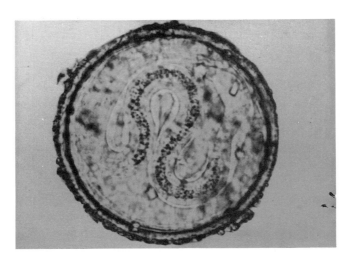

**Fig. 7.2**   Eggs of *Parascaris equorum*.

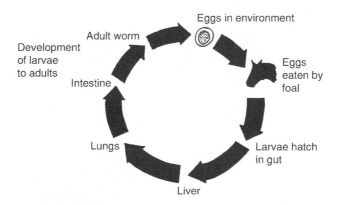

**Fig. 7.3** Life cycle of ascarid.

passed out in the foal's droppings and thus infecting the pasture. From the eggs being passed out of the foal in the dung to the development of infective larvae takes about 30 days under optimal conditions.

Foals may have up to 1000 adult ascarids in their gut, giving them a dull coat, pot-belly, loss of condition and slow growth. The worms will cause inflammation of the lining of the gut and in severe cases may actually block the small intestine, causing rupture, peritonitis and death. The migrating larvae can cause coughing and a snotty nose.

Very heavy contamination can occur on paddocks grazed every year by mares and foals. Mares must be wormed regularly during pregnancy, and ideally foals should only be turned out on to pasture that has not been grazed by a horse in the previous 12 months.

After the age of two horses develop resistance to ascarids, and they do not cause problems in older horses.

### Threadworms *(Strongyloides westeri)*

This parasite of foals can be passed from the mare via her milk or can enter the foal by penetrating the foal's skin (Fig. 7.4). The adults live in the small intestine and are very small and generally well tolerated. However heavy infection can cause scouring in foals two to four weeks old, which may coincide with the mare's foaling heat. Foals can be treated for threadworm from seven days old but regular worming of the mare will help reduce the incidence and severity of threadworm infection (Fig. 7.5). Infection is rarely seen in youngstock more than six months old. Threadworms are difficult to control with conventional wormers, requiring high dosage or the use of ivermectin.

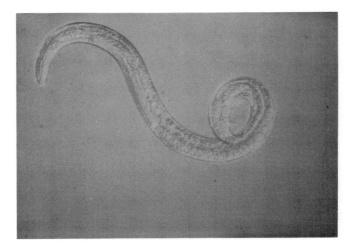

**Fig. 7.4**  *Strongyloides westeri* – free living adult.

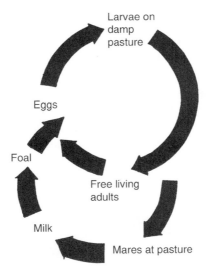

**Fig. 7.5**  Life cycle of *Strongloides westeri*.

## Large strongyles *(Strongylus vulgaris & S. edentatus)* **and small** strongyles *(Trichonema species)*

These are the most important parasites of horses, affecting horses of all ages. Large strongyles are round worms, between 2 and 8 cm (1–3 inches) long and coloured red from the blood that they suck, while small stron-

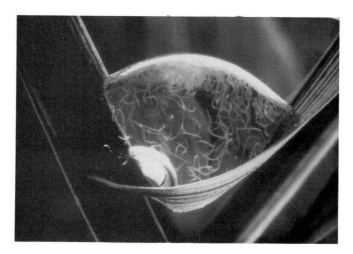

**Fig. 7.6**   Small strongyle.

gyles are greyish white round worms 0.5 to 2.5 cm ($\frac{1}{4}$ – 1 inch) in length (Fig. 7.6). They are divided into two main groups but the life-cycles are similar; eggs are laid by the adult worm in the large intestine and passed out in the droppings (Fig. 7.7).

Although fewer eggs are produced by strongyles than by ascarids the eggs can remain viable on the paddock until late May or early June of the following year. The larvae develop on the grass and become infective third stage (L3) larvae; the speed of this development depends upon the

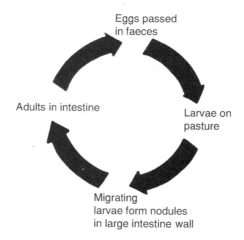

**Fig. 7.7**   Life cycle of small strongyle.

climate and takes about 10 days in warm, moist conditions. The L3 larvae are eaten by the grazing horse and pass into the intestines. Here the life-cycles vary: small strongyles burrow into the wall of the large intestine and emerge two to three months later as egg-laying adults (Figs. 7.8 and 7.9). These larvae can remain dormant for many months, making them difficult to control using many wormers. This shorter life-cycle means that several generations of larvae will be passed out in one grazing season, and

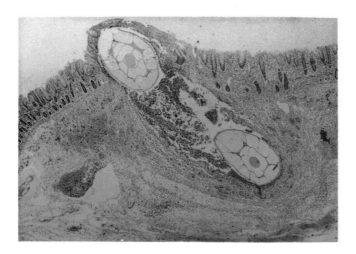

**Fig. 7.8**  Small strongyle in lining of gut.

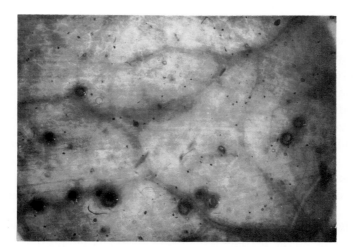

**Fig. 7.9**  Small strongyles in gut lining.

consequently pasture contamination can become very heavy indeed, leading to high worm burdens in the horse.

Small redworm have become increasingly important due to their life-cycle and the development of resistance to the benzimidazole group of wormers. In the autumn, the larvae burrow into the wall of the gut and become encysted, remaining dormant for many months. During this time few wormers are active against them and then only effective in high doses. This means that it is important to have an effective worming programme throughout the year to keep the population of developing larvae at low levels, so that as few larvae as possible become encysted in the autumn. In the late winter or spring (December to May) encysted larvae are triggered to continue their development and emerge into the gut. Large numbers entering the gut may cause:

- weight loss
- diarrhoea
- sluggish behaviour
- loss of appetite
- colic
- filled legs
- fever
- dehydration.

Controlling redworm infection involves:

- Regular worming during the grazing season to control the number of egg-laying adults and hence the number of infective larvae on the pasture.
- Annual testing of the horses droppings for the presence of worm eggs to ensure the worming programme is effective. This is particularly important if the benzimidazole wormers have been used.
- Changing to a chemically unrelated wormer every year to avoid the buildup of resistance.
- A five-day course of fenbendazole will remove encysted larvae and should be used to treat a horse whose worming history is unknown.
- The manufacturers recommend a five-day course in November to remove larvae picked up in the summer and another course in February to remove any larvae which have encysted over the winter.

*S. vulgaris* migrates extensively through the body: about eight days after infection the larvae become fourth stage (L4) larvae and migrate to the anterior mesenteric artery, responsible for supplying most of the gut with

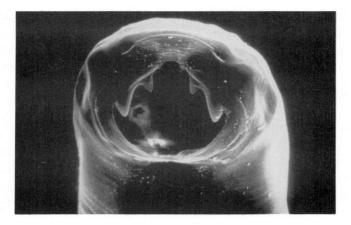

**Fig. 7.10**  Mouthparts of *S. vulgaris.*

blood (Fig. 7.10). This migration damages the artery walls (aneurysms) and causes blood clots, which may block smaller blood vessels and thus disrupt the blood supply to the gut causing colic. Indeed redworm are thought to be the commonest cause of recurrent bouts of spasmodic colic. Eventually the mature larvae return to the wall of the large intestine before emerging into the gut where they become egg-laying adults five to nine months after infection.

The larvae of *S. edentatus* penetrate the wall of the large intestine and migrate through the liver to the lining of the abdomen. Larvae return to the wall of the large intestine, form nodules and subsequently emerge to become egg-laying adults 5–12 months after being eaten by the horse. The nodular larval stages consume blood and cause digestive upsets while the adults cause irritation and ulcers by feeding on the gut wall.

This prolonged migration may lead to 'false negative' faecal worm egg counts. There may be no adult egg-laying worms in the gut, and thus a negative worm egg count will be recorded, even though the tissues may contain many larvae which are causing extensive damage and which will eventually become adults in the gut. Both large and small strongyles can remain dormant in the gut wall, so that when egg-laying adults are removed by worming, a new wave of larvae emerge and become egg-laying adults. This is known as larval cyathostomiasis and tends to be most obvious in the spring. Few wormers are active against these migrating larvae, though some are effective in high doses; it is wise to give a larvicidal dose at intervals through the year to reduce the population of developing larvae.

Redworms can affect horses of all ages. Foals less than six weeks old will not harbour any egg laying adults but the larval stages will start to cause damage soon after being eaten.

## Pinworms *(Oxyuris equi, seatworm)*

Pinworms are white round worms between 1 and 10 cm ($\frac{1}{4}$ – 4 inches) long and 1 mm ($\frac{1}{25}$ inch) in diameter; they are killed by routine doses of wormer and are not usually a problem. The adults live in the large intestine, and the female lays her eggs on the skin surrounding the anus, which causes intense itching. Larvae develop in the egg within four days, and the eggs then fall on the pasture where the grazing horse eats them. After ingestion the larvae hatch and develop in the wall of the large intestine before becoming egg-laying adults four to five months later. Eggs can remain viable for 12 months on pasture.

## Bots *(Gasterophilus spp)*

The bee-like adult bot fly lays its yellow eggs on the hairs of the horse's legs, shoulders and neck during the summer months, from July to September. When the horse licks itself it takes eggs into its mouth; the eggs hatch and the maggot-like larvae pass to the stomach, where the larvae mature before being passed out in the droppings eight to ten months later in the following spring (Fig. 7.11). The larvae pupate and

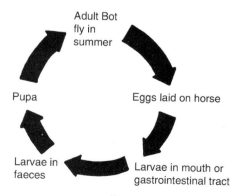

**Fig. 7.11**  Life cycle of bot.

then hatch three to five weeks later as adult flies to complete the cycle. Traditionally horses have been treated for bots in the late autumn, after the first frosts, and again in the spring to remove any bots that did not pass out spontaneously. Large bot populations can cause ulceration of the horse's stomach.

## Lungworm (Dictyocaulus arnfieldi)

Lungworm can cause acute coughing, but even badly affected horses may not pass out eggs or larvae in the droppings. This makes diagnosis of lungworm difficult; indeed diagnosis may only follow successful treatment.

## Tapeworm (Anoplocephala perfoliata)

The adult tapeworm (Fig. 7.12) is found in the caecum and favours the ileocaecal junction, where the small intestine enters the caecum. The adult is segmented and about 8 cm (3 inches) long and 8–14 mm ($\frac{1}{4}$ – $\frac{1}{2}$ inch) wide; it sheds segments containing eggs which are passed out in the dung. Eggs are eaten by an intermediate host, forage mites, where larval development takes place (Fig. 7.13). The horse is infected by eating these mites while grazing, and the larval form develops directly to the adult

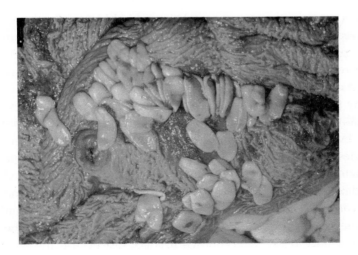

**Fig. 7.12**   Tapeworm.

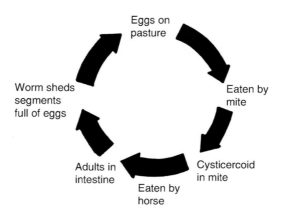

**Fig. 7.13**  Life cycle of tapeworm.

worm in the caecum, taking six to ten weeks. Infection has been associated with colics, peritonitis and digestive upsets due to inflammation of the gut around the area of attachment. There are a few wormers which are effective against tapeworms, and it may be advisable to treat foals and adult horses (excluding stallions and pregnant mares) once or twice a year with an effective wormer.

## Treatment and control

Correct and efficient use of anthelmintics or wormers is vital to good stable and grassland management; horses should be wormed every four to six weeks in order to suppress worm egg output and to minimise the migrating larval stages in the tissues. This applies equally to the pony out all year round and to the eventer or racehorse that only has short spells out at grass.

In any parasite control programme there should be a changeover to a chemically-unrelated wormer every 12 months in order to prevent the worms building up a resistance to one product (see Table 7.3). Small strongyles have been shown to develop resistance to wormers containing the benzimidazole group of chemicals: this group includes fenbendazole, mebendazole, febantel, oxibendazole, oxfendazole and thiabendazole. Once worms have developed resistance to one of the benzimidazole group they commonly show resistance to other wormers from the same group and once resistance is shown it is not lost even if the wormer is changed. This means that benzimidazole wormers should be avoided

**Table 7.3**  Drugs available for control of internal parasites.

| Trade name | Manufacturer | Active ingredient |
|---|---|---|
| *Benzimidazole drugs for roundworms* | | |
| Panacur | Hoechst | Fenbendazole |
| Telmin | Janssen Pharmaceutical | Mebendazole |
| Equizole | Mereck Sharp & Dohme | Thiabendazole |
| Equitac | Smith Kline | Oxibendazole |
| Systamex | Wellcome | Oxfendazole |
| *Other compounds for roundworms* | | |
| Pony and foal wormer | Crown Chemicals | Piperazine |
| Strongid-P | Pfizer | Pyrantel embonate |
| Pyratape-P | Hoechst Roussel Vet | Pyrantel embonate |
| Eqvalan | Merck Sharp & Dohme | Ivermectin |
| Furexel | Jansson | Ivermectin |
| Equest | Fort Doge Animal Health Ltd | Moxidectin |
| *Benzimidazole drugs for encysted small redworm* | | |
| Panacur Guard | Hoechst | Fenbendazole |
| *Organic phosphorus compounds for bot-fly larvae* | | |
| Neguvon | Bayer | Trichlorfon |
| Equigard | Shell Chemicals | Dichlorvos |

permanently. It is important to have a dung sample analysed once a year. If you have wormed regularly as advised, and yet the horse is still passing out large numbers of eggs, it is likely that the worms have become resistant to the chemical in the product that you are using. Resistance is more likely to occur if all the horses on a yard have been wormed frequently with a benzimidazole wormer, particularly if the paddocks are 'horse sick'.

Good grassland management will help control the free-living stage of the parasites; appropriate techniques include ploughing and reseeding, rest and rotation, removal of droppings, harrowing and topping. Paddocks should not be overstocked with horses and grazing with sheep and cattle will help reduce pasture contamination.

All horses should be wormed prior to turn out and before introducing them to fresh pasture. It is recommended that all horses grazing the same field are wormed at the same time. Regular worming is most important when the weather is warm and damp as these are ideal conditions for

**Table 7.4**  Which wormer to use.

| Parasite | Drug/Wormer | Comment |
|---|---|---|
| Routine worming for adult large and small strongyles (will also kill pinworm) | Fenbendazole (Panacur) Ivermectin (Eqvalan) Mebendazole (Telmin) Oxfendazole (Systamex) Piperazine (various) Thiabendazole (Equizole) Pyrantel (Strongid-P) | Does not kill the eggs |
| Migrating strongyle larvae | Fenbendazole (Panacur) Ivermectin (Eqvalan) Oxfendazole (Systamex)  Fenbendazole | One dose a day for 5 days Effective at normal level 50 per cent effective at normal level Five-day course |
| Encysted strongyle larvae | Moxidectin | Normal dose |
| *Strongyloides westeri* in foals: 1–4 weeks | Ivermectin (Eqvalan) Thiabendazole (Equizole) Fenbendazole (Panacur) | Requires high dose; 25 ml Panacur 10 per cent or half syringe |
| Ascarids in foals: from four weeks to eight months dose every four weeks | Ivermectin (Eqvalan) Pyrantel (Strongid-P) Fenbendazole (Panacur) Oxfendazole (Systamex) Mebendazole (Telmin) | High dose rate needed |
| Lungworm | Ivermectin (Eqvalan) Fenbendazole (Panacur) Mebendazole (Telmin) | High dose daily for five days |
| Bots | Ivermectin (Eqvalan) Dichlorvos (Equigard) Trichlorfon (Neguvon) | Also effective against strongyles, pinworm and ascarids |
| Tapeworm | Pyrantel embonate | Requires double dose |

large numbers of larvae to hatch from the eggs on the grass. A wormer active against bots should be incorporated into the programme at the appropriate time.

# Colic

Colic is not a disease but an abdominal pain which may be caused by a wide variety of disorders. The primary cause of this pain is distension of the stomach or intestines which may be due to an accumulation of gas, fluid or feed caused by a blockage or improper movement of the gut. Generally the vet should be called as soon as colic is suspected; hay and feed should be removed and the horse left alone, unless it is so violent as to be in danger of injuring itself, in which case it should be walked and kept warm.

## Spasmodic colic

Spasmodic colic is caused by spasm of the muscular wall of the intestine; there may be several reasons for this including damage to the intestinal wall by migrating strongyle larvae, or feeding and drinking too soon after fast work. Affected horses are usually moderately distressed, showing signs of sweating and constantly going down and getting up. They may look at and kick at their flanks and roll, often getting cast. The pulse rate may rise to 68–92 beats per minute and will be over 100 in severe cases; similarly the respiration rate will increase up to 80 per minute and the temperature will go up. They usually pass few droppings but the condition may come and go quite quickly. If it persists treatment with a relaxant drug usually relieves the problem rapidly.

## Impactive colic

Impactive colics account for about 30 per cent of all colics and are caused by impaction of food material in the large intestine. This often occurs at the pelvic flexure where the intestine narrows near the pelvis to turn back towards the chest. It may occur because the horse has eaten its bedding, or when it is brought in from grass and goes onto a hay ration. Affected horses are not usually in a great deal of pain and tend to look dull and off-colour, getting up and down in an uncomfortable manner and rolling more than usual. The vet will insert his hand into the horse's rectum to try and feel where the blockage is; he may give it pain killers and also large amounts of liquid paraffin, or a similar agent, via a stomach tube to stimulate gut movement.

## Distension (tympanic) colic

Distension colic is caused by a buildup of gas in the gut and is usually very painful; horses will sweat and roll violently, often hurting themselves in the process. Gas buildup may occur in front of an impaction, may be due to a twist in the gut, or be caused by fermentation of food in the stomach or small intestine.

## Intestinal catastrophe

Commonly known as twisted gut, this is the most dramatic and serious form of colic. The intestine becomes twisted, telescoped into itself or rotated about its mesentary, all of which obstruct the blood supply. Horses become uncontrollably violent in their agony and immediate veterinary attention is vital if the horse is to survive, as abdominal surgery is necessary.

## Predisposing factors for colic

- Sudden access to large quantities of rich feed e.g. grass clippings, cereals, fallen apples, lush grass.
- Changed routine, new stable, new surroundings.
- Irregular work, changes in feeding routine.
- Working on full stomach.
- Exhaustion.
- Feeding and/or watering too soon after fast work.
- Mouldy feed.
- Sudden change of diet.
- Sharp teeth.
- Greedy feeders.

## Prevention of colic

As with most problems good stable management and correct feeding are the answer:

- Feed each horse as an individual, noting its idiosyncrasies.
- Feed concentrates little and often, keeping to regular feeding times – even at weekends.
- Make changes to the diet gradually; do not increase concentrates by more than 0.5 kg a day when building up a ration.
- Have a planned, regular exercise programme.
- Feed good quality feed and store it away from vermin.
- Keep to your routine, even when away from home.
- Cool the horse thoroughly after strenuous work before allowing it to drink and eat large amounts.
- Have the teeth checked and rasped regularly.
- Stop horses bolting their feed by adding chaff or putting a salt lick or large stones in the manger.
- Keep to a regular effective worming programme.

## Enteritis

Enteritis is inflammation of the intestines marked by diarrhoea or scouring. It can occur in any age or type of horse and is due to poor feeding, parasites or bacterial or viral infection. Overfeeding with very high protein feeds, a sudden change of feed and mouldy feed can all cause problems. The horse should be fed only hay and water until the diarrhoea clears up; if the symptoms persist the vet should check the horse for parasites or infection.

In severe cases the horse will need fluid intravenously to replace that lost when scouring, so that it does not become dehydrated. Foals are particularly susceptible to dehydration.

## Azoturia

Despite intensive investigation azoturia (tying up, setfast, exertional rhabdomyolysis, Monday morning disease) remains a poorly-understood disease resulting in muscle stiffness and pain; it can occur under different circumstances and to a variable degree. Traditionally the problem arises soon after the onset of exercise, particularly in fit horses, maintained on a full ration, the day after a rest day. The signs vary from slight hind leg stiffness to severe pain and total reluctance to move. However horses have been known to develop symptoms at grass in the ten minute box of a three-day event or during walking exercise. Some horses are prone to recurrent attacks and highly-strung horses, especially mares, are susceptible. Vitamin E and/or selenium have been implicated but there is little information to support this and opinion seems to suggest an electrolyte imbalance as being a key point.

Whatever the cause the result is muscle damage, releasing muscle enzymes into the blood stream; these enzymes (CPK and AST) are used to assess the severity of the attack and the speed at which the levels in the blood fall is used to monitor the rate of recovery from an attack. Lactic acid is also released from the damaged muscle cells, and continuing to work a mildly affected horse can make the condition much worse; it is vital to stop work immediately and get the horse back to his box with as little energy expenditure as possible.

Treatment involves reduction of pain and inflammation; the horse may need to be sedated and have fluid therapy and it is important to keep him warm. The horse should have only hay and water plus any medicines prescribed by the vet. Prevention is through careful stable management and attention to diet.

- Cut the concentrates if the horse has a day off.
- Warm up and cool the horse down properly.
- Make sure that the diet contains adequate calcium, phosphorus and salt (sodium chloride).
- Find a low energy, low protein feed, for example horse and pony cubes, that suits your horse.

# Laminitis

Laminitis can be a life-threatening condition and prevention is infinitely better than cure.

## Anatomy of the foot

The force created by the horse's weight is transmitted down through the bones of the leg to the pedal bone, which sits within the hoof wall; the force is then transferred to the hoof wall and then to the ground. The pedal bone (and therefore the horse's weight) is suspended from the inside of the hoof wall by two interleaving sets of laminae.

One set of laminae project out as thin sheets of tissue from the pedal bone and the second set project inwards from the hoof wall. Main laminae are called primary laminae, each of which has many secondary laminae projecting from its surface. This results in an increase in the surface area bonding the outside of the bone and the inside of the wall and reduces the stress across the junction. The laminar junction contains specialised blood vessels known as arterio-venous anastomoses (AVAs) which allow blood to pass rapidly from arteries to veins without passing through the small blood vessels (capillaries) of the foot. AVAs probably act as pressure-relief valves so that the capillaries do not burst when the foot hits the ground.

## What is laminitis?

Laminitis is a weakening or destruction of the laminae, thought to result from lack of blood supply to the affected region. The development of the disease is not completely understood and other mechanisms may be involved. Mild cases of laminitis may go unnoticed, with no permanent damage to the foot. In more severe cases, the lack of blood supply causes the laminae on the outside of the bone to detach from the laminae on the inside of the hoof wall. In the worst cases, the weakened laminar junction can no longer support the weight of the horse, and the pedal bone moves within the hoof and may penetrate the sole of the foot.

## Causes of laminitis

Occasionally a horse or pony will get laminitis for no obvious reason; however, the factors listed below all significantly increase the chances of an animal becoming affected.

- Excessive feed intake: ponies allowed unrestricted access to pasture, particularly lush spring grass, are at extremely high risk. Grass intake should be strictly limited in these circumstances, the aim being to maintain ideal body weight. Extreme care should be taken if concentrates are fed to ponies, and thought should be given to eliminating them from the diet completely in high-risk animals. 'Overfeeding' laminitis can also occur in horses, where it is most commonly due to excessive concentrate intake. The classic case is the horse which escapes and gains access to the feed bin.
- Toxemia: horses which have toxins in their bloodstream are at high risk of laminitis. Common causes of toxemia are severe diarrhoea, pleuritis, some types of severe colic and retention of the placenta (afterbirth) after foaling.
- Trauma: laminitis occasionally occurs in horses or ponies which exercise excessively on very hard ground.
- Excessive weight-bearing: horses which are very lame in one leg may develop laminitis in the opposite leg due to excessive weight-bearing.
- Steroids: corticosteroids can cause laminitis and should never be used to treat laminitis.
- Cushings disease or cancer of the pituitary gland: the most obvious signs are excessive drinking and development of an excessively long coat. These animals are prone to laminitis.

## Signs of laminitis

The signs of laminitis vary from mild lameness visible only at a trot, to an animal that stands rooted to the spot, refusing to move, to one that is down and blowing in pain. The main signs are listed below:

- varying degree of lameness
- reluctance to move, standing with hind feet under body and fore feet stretched out in front
- prominent, bounding digital arterial pulse
- hot feet, horses feet normally heat up and cool down during the course of a day but marked heat in the feet for several hours may indicate laminitis

*What to do*

The vet should be called immediately, in the mean time:

- The horse should not be allowed to eat anything or given any drugs.
- If the horse can walk reasonably easily, it should be put in a deeply bedded stable.
- It is important that the horse is not walked any further or faster than necessary. Forced walking of animals with laminitis is now known to be extremely detrimental.

## Prevention

Prevention of laminitis revolves around careful horse management:

- do not allow horses, and particularly ponies, to become overweight
- restrict grass intake when grass is lush and plentiful
- never overfeed concentrate feed
- keep concentrates in horse-proof containers
- provide skilled, regular foot care.

## Feed-related laminitis

An overload of carbohydrates such as sugars and starches can result in undigested soluble carbohydrate reaching the hind gut. These sugars and starches are fermented far more quickly than the fibre in hay, coarse grass and chaff, resulting in the bacteria producing VFAs more quickly than they can be absorbed. The end result is a buildup of acid in the hind gut which appears to be one of the triggers of laminitis. Acid buildup can be prevented by controlling the diet and minimising the intake of starch and sugars.

*Sugars in grass*

Grass forms a major part of the diet for most horses and ponies. Grass stores carbohydrates as starch (10–13 per cent) and sugars (up to 90 per cent). These sugars are made up of sucrose and a group of higher homologues of sucrose known as 'fructans'. Sucrose and fructan are known as water-soluble carbohydrates (WSC) and the concentrations in grass can vary dramatically within hours, with levels equivalent to 5–50 per cent of total dry matter. High fructan levels in grass have been linked to the onset of laminitis and an understanding of when and how the fructan levels may be high will help in the management of the laminitic horse or pony.

The amount of WSC in grass will depend on:

- how much is being made
- how much is being used by the plant
- the recent history of the plant, i.e. has the supply of WSC been greater than the demand, allowing the accumulation of WSC.

Fructans tend to be high where growth is reduced; thus stress conditions such as severe grazing, low temperature and low soil fertility result in the accumulation of fructan. Many factors are involved in determining the amount of WSC in grass, making it difficult to predict how much WSC there will be in the sward at any one time.

### Digestion of fructan

While sucrose is digested in the small intestine, fructan is fermented in the hind gut along with dietary fibre. Fructans are readily but selectively utilised by certain microbial species, at the expense of others. In human and pig nutrition fructans are regarded as being beneficial but it would appear that large amounts of fructans, for example in spring grass on a sunny day, lead to rapid and major changes to the environment of the horse's hind gut. This results in the proliferation of some species and the death of others; it is the release of toxins by these dying bacteria that is implicated in the onset of laminitis.

### Practical management of grassland

There are so many factors involved in determining the level of fructan in grass that it is not possible to recommend a safe time to turn out to grass, horses and ponies that are susceptible to laminitis. The only way to remove the risk is to keep the animal stabled during the growing season and feed low-fructan forages; for example, hay made from mature grass or alfalfa. Extra energy can be supplied by adding sunflower or soya oil to chaff and a mineral and vitamin supplement should also be fed.

In the future it may be possible to cultivate pastures of low WSC species of grasses and legumes, which with careful management could be grazed by the laminitic. It is hoped that methods will be developed to predict the WSC and fructan level of the grass so that owners can decide if it is 'safe' to turn horses and ponies out to grass.

*Acknowledgement*

This section on Laminitis has been taken from the proceedings of the Dodson and Horrell International Conference on Equine Laminitis (1998).

# Lymphangitis

The lymphatic system is a network of fine tubes which collect excess fluid from all parts of the body and return it to the blood stream; the return of lymph is aided by muscle massage. Too little exercise and excess feeding lead to the waterlogging in the tissues and consequently the area becomes swollen. This oedema pits when firm pressure is applied. The lack of exercise means reduced muscle massage, making it more difficult to return the lymph; the rich food disturbs the delicate protein and electrolyte balance and the lymph system is unable to carry away the waste material and excess fluid.

The legs may become filled when the walls of the blood and lymph vessels are damaged by toxins, so that water passes into the tissue spaces very quickly. The damage may be due to an allergic reaction to a feed or a drug, or may be a direct result of a viral or bacterial infection. Diets high in protein may aggravate the swelling due to the nutritional element adding to the drainage problem.

Lymphangitis usually occurs in the hind limb and may lead to a permanently enlarged limb. Treatment aims to combat infection and relieve pain so that controlled exercise can be given. The amount and type of feed must be looked at and changed if necessary.

# Developmental Orthopaedic Disease (DOD)

The amount and composition of the feed in a young, growing horse's diet is vital in determining correct growth and development; unlike farm stock, which are grown as quickly as possible, we have to make sure that horses grow in such a way that their athletic ability is not affected. Developmental Orthopaedic Disease (DOD) is a general term for a number of problems that arise in growing horses. Many of these are related to nutrition, for example epiphysitis, 'contracted tendons', 'wobblers', bone cysts, and osteochondrosis. These are all serious conditions and veterinary advice should be sought in all cases.

## *Epiphysitis*

This refers to pain associated with abnormal activity in a growth plate; usually the lower growth plate of the radius, just above the knee or in the fetlock area, at the end of the cannon bone. It occurs in young, rapidly-growing horses, most commonly yearlings but foals can also be affected. There is usually swelling and heat just above the knee; the horse may or may not be lame but there is often pain if pressure is applied to the area. Where the condition is slight it will resolve itself but if severe the diet should be restricted to good quality hay and the youngster confined to the stable until the swellings go down. Foals may have their milk intake limited. This restriction in diet will slow the growth rate so that the joints can 'catch up' and mature without excess strain. Once the bumps have subsided there should be light exercise daily and a gradual increase in diet back to normal.

Epiphysitis can develop in less than a week and immediate treatment is important to aid successful recovery. Prevention is even better and energy and protein intake must be controlled and a correct mineral and trace element balance maintained.

## *Contracted tendons (flexor tendon deformities)*

Contracted tendons can be present at birth (congenital) or develop after birth (acquired). Rapidly-growing foals between six weeks and six months are most commonly affected by acquired flexor tendon deformities, the condition appearing in one or both front limbs. The foal may stand high on its toes at birth, in which case it should be exercised regularly and allowed to grow slowly, or it may be seen to 'go up on its toes'; the limb becomes more upright and the foot becomes boxy. As soon as the condition is spotted (and it may occur very suddenly) the foal's growth rate must be slowed by cutting out any supplementary feed and restricting the mare's feed for three or four weeks. If this is carefully monitored there should not be an effect on the foal's mature size. The feet must be trimmed to lower the heels as much as possible, and it may be necessary to have the foal shod until the condition resolves.

## *'Wobblers'*

The wobbler syndrome describes a number of conditions that lead to compression of the spinal cord in the neck causing a typical uncoordinated gait. The clinical signs may be sudden and severe or subtle and insidious in onset. The horse may show intermittent hind leg lameness, and as the condition worsens the horse will tend to stand with its hind legs in odd positions and become less coordinated. The syndrome occurs most commonly in young, rapidly-growing horses; high planes of nutrition which encourage this rapid growth should be avoided so that the young horse is allowed to grow more slowly.

## Osteochondrosis (OCD)

Osteochondrosis (OCD) is abnormal development of cartilage and bone, found most commonly in young, rapidly-growing horses. There may be a genetic predisposition to the disease in foals bred to grow quickly; the high planes of nutrition often fed to these foals may increase the risk of the condition occurring. The disease is most often found in the stifle, hock and shoulder joints.

As bone grows and develops, cartilage is turned into bone, and if this conversion is delayed by a poor blood supply then the cartilage on the joint surface becomes abnormally thick, and the lower layers of cartilage may die. This means that the cartilage is only loosely attached to the underlying bone and may detach, causing inflammation and pain.

## Bone cysts

Bone cysts are holes in the bone close to the joint surface. The condition may be related to OCD but the exact cause is not known. It is important to take veterinary advice on the treatment of OCD and bone cysts.

## The incidence of DOD

The incidence of DOD fluctuates and appears to be related to grass supply and hence climatic conditions. For example, the patterns of grass growth in 1989 and 1990 were very unusual and the extremes of weather played havoc with the normal seasonal variations in quality and quantity of pasture. The winter of 1989–90 was mild and because many paddocks still had plenty of grass, many young horses were left out. In addition in-foal mares received little, if any supplementary feed because they were keeping their condition and the grass appeared to be providing adequate nutrients. The spring of 1990 had a greater than usual incidence of DOD, so it was decided that pasture analysis should begin earlier in the year to try and establish if grass quality was having an effect. It was found that many pastures had extremely unbalanced mineral levels, with levels of some essential minerals being very low. Several trends emerged from this work:

(1) In early spring, when many yearlings are beginning a growth spurt, calcium levels were very low in some areas. In extreme cases the calcium levels were lower than those of phosphorus. This meant that unless additional calcium was fed to the youngstock to restore the calcium: phosphorus ratio then those young horses were not getting adequate nutrients for growth.

(2) The spring sees the foetus inside the pregnant mare making the majority of its growth, needing high levels of calcium for bone growth. Both the mares and their developing foals were low in calcium, and it is thought that certain bone abnormalities can occur while the foetus is still developing.

(3) Magnesium levels were also low: magnesium forms nearly 1 per cent of the mineral matrix of the skeleton, so low levels will obviously have an effect on bone quality.

(4) The importance of copper in the maturation of bone has been researched and it is believed that low dietary copper is significant in DOD. In 1990 the copper levels were also very low, and this was made worse by high levels of sulphur interfering with copper uptake. Molybdenum will also make copper less available to the grazing horse.

(5) Zinc, another important mineral in bone development, was also very low in grass.

Remember that the hay made from this grass will also have all these deficiencies and imbalances and so the situation will continue through the following winter.

Protein and energy levels in pasture will also affect the growth and development of youngstock: high levels will result in them getting fat and putting strain on young limbs and joints. They may also grow too quickly and this, along with the imbalances already mentioned, increases the chances of growth problems arising. The provision of mineral supplements to youngstock and broodmares is vital, especially if the grass is meeting the energy and protein requirements so that they are not receiving any concentrate feed.

# Allergies

Urticaria, hives and nettlerash are common allergies; the natural response of the skin to allergic reactions may be the sudden appearance of variable sized lumps. Animal proteins in concentrate feeds and fresh grass proteins often produce an allergic reaction. The horse develops many small, firm bumps on the body which may be very itchy and the horse may go off its feed. Old-fashioned books called this condition 'surfeit'.

# Obesity and overfeeding

We have discussed some of the results of overfeeding both young and adult horses, but there are a number of other consequences:

(1) Overfed horses will become obese, a condition as undesirable in horses as it is in humans. Obesity is said to reduce fertility of mares and certainly can make foaling more difficult. Fat horses cannot work as efficiently, the respiratory system, tendons, joints and ligaments will all be put under greater strain and the horse will become fatigued more quickly.

(2) Fat horses that are suddenly deprived of food may get hyperlipaemia (as described in the section on laminitis); pony mares in late pregnancy or early lactation that experience a sudden change in pasture are prone to this problem.

(3) Young horses kept in yards and fed as a group often have one aggressive individual that eats more than the others. This may cause enterotoxaemia, a flatulent colic which occurs because the intestines are overloaded with rich feed, leading to gas build-up. There may also be signs of laboured breathing and swelling under the skin, apparently due to the bacterium *Clostridium perfringens* proliferating. This is a normal inhabitant of the gut that secretes an enterotoxin; the horse can cope with this toxin in small amounts but large amounts cause damage to the intestine wall and start diarrhoea.

# Acidosis

Acidosis occurs when there is a buildup of acid (hydrogen ions) in the blood and body tissues. Respiratory acidosis is caused by the retention of carbon dioxide by the lungs; metabolic acidosis occurs when there is a high level of lactic acid.

# Dehydration

Dehydration is excessive loss of water from the body tissues and may follow prolonged sweating in working horses or severe diarrhoea in horses suffering from salmonella infection or strongyle infection. The adult horse's body is approximately 65–75 per cent water and the foal is 75–80 per cent water; water is vital for life, and any excess loss of water is bound to have serious consequences. The horse does not only lose water but also important electrolytes, including sodium, potassium and chloride. These electrolytes are involved in maintaining the correct volume and water content of the body cells, and the horse must keep the cellular levels of these minerals within strict limits if he is to stay healthy. Any loss of fluids and electrolytes must be made good rapidly, especially in young stock as dehydration can kill surprisingly rapidly.

After work dehydrated horses should be given about 4.5 litres (1 gallon) of water every 15 minutes, containing 30 g (1 oz) electrolytes. If the horse will not drink, electrolyte replacement may be intravenous or via a stomach tube, using an electrolyte solution containing sodium chloride (common salt), glucose, lactate, potassium, calcium and magnesium; your veterinary surgeon will advise you. If the dehydration is mild then electrolytes in the water or feed for several days may be adequate. Electrolytes do not need to be fed unless the horse is or is likely to become dehydrated; unnecessarily high levels of these minerals may be harmful.

Horses should be allowed to drink often during long periods of work. If the weather is very hot then two minutes drinking every two hours is indicated; this way the horse will take water little and often. Large amounts of water may be harmful and the working horse is only able to utilise small drinks efficiently.

# Chapter 8
# Practical Feeding

No matter how good your knowledge of anatomy, physiology and food science, you still have to be able to make an educated, instant decision on what to feed a horse as soon as it walks onto the yard. This chapter gives guidelines on practical feeding by linking the art and the science of feeding horses.

## Rules of feeding – update

- Feed by weight not volume.
- Feed to fitness required.
- Feed to just below appetite.
- Feed lots of roughage and as few concentrates as possible.
- Feed to bodyweight, taking the horse's condition into account.
- Adjust and alter the ration as necessary – you must be happy with what you are feeding.
- Worm regularly.
- Check the teeth regularly.

*Feed by weight not volume*

Traditionally concentrates have been fed by the scoop, in other words by volume. If asked what we feed our horses most of us would reply in terms of scoops, and have very little idea of the number of pounds that would weigh, let alone how many kilograms. The energy and other nutrients provided are dependent on the weight fed – your feed scoop should be marked to show the volume occupied by 1 kg or 1 lb of the types of feed that you use. Use the kitchen scales and some insulating tape to calibrate your scoop. For the purposes of Table 8.1 I have assumed that a 'scoop' holds 2 litres; your scoop may be different but it serves to illustrate that if you substitute one scoop of barley for oats you will be overfeeding your

**Table 8.1**  Energy values of some common horse feeds.

| Feed | Digestible energy (MJ per kg dry matter) | Digestible energy (MJ per 'scoop') |
|------|------------------------------------------|-------------------------------------|
| Oats | 11–12 | 10 |
| Barley | 13 | 15 |
| Maize | 14 | 19 |
| Extracted soyabean meal | 13.3 | 17 |
| Wheatbran | 11 | 5 |

horse 5 MJ DE. This is not only going to have an effect on your horse, but also on your pocket; imagine that overfeeding being multiplied for every day of the year.

Forage should also be weighed: how many people know what a 5 lb haynet looks like? Horses are fed hay in 'slices' or 'wedges', which can vary dramatically from bale to bale. It is good practice and worth the extra time (until you get your eye in) to hang a small spring balance in the hay barn and weigh the horse's haynet so that you know he is getting what you calculated with the rules of rationing and not being overfed. A major cause of horses becoming fussy and not eating up is simply overfeeding.

As a rule of thumb an average bale weighs 20–25 kg (44–55 lb). A 500 kg horse on a maintenance ration and being fed average quality hay needs only 8–9 kg (18–20 lb) of hay a day. This is only one-third of a bale of hay. It is no wonder that horses on box-rest and being fed to appetite to stop them getting bored often put on weight.

### Feed to fitness required

Plan your horse's feeding and fitness regime together; they go hand in hand. Overfeeding is just as bad as underfeeding and probably more dangerous to you and your horse.

### Feed to just below appetite

If a horse is always fed as much as he can eat, he will eventually become sated and go off his feed. If he is fed a little below his appetite he will always be ready for his next feed of hay or concentrates.

### Feed as few concentrates as possible

Concentrates are not a natural feed for horses, and in excess contribute to problems such as azoturia, lymphangitis and laminitis. The more fibre the horse receives, the healthier his gut will be and the happier the 'bugs' that break down the fibre. Very often as horses get fit they tend to ration themselves, and many racehorses and eventers are fed as much hay as they want and do not get a 'belly'. A problem may arise with the moderately fit horse, like the dressage horse; he is not doing fast work and does not ration himself and will get fat at the drop of a hat. The same is true of good 'doers': these horses may need to have their hay rationed but providing that you balance the ratio of forage to concentrate properly and then weigh both hay and concentrates, you should be able to keep the horse both happy and slim.

## Feeding the in-foal broodmare

The in-foal mare should be kept as naturally as possible so that she stays relaxed, happy and healthy. Overfeeding is detrimental to the mare's health and the subsequent condition of the newborn foal.

### Summer to Christmas

From the time she is tested in-foal until October, good quality pasture should satisfy all her nutrient requirements. Mares need to be kept fit not fat: the mare's ribs should not be visible but they should be easily detected on touch, with no thick layer of fat disguising them. This will make foaling easier and enhance her chances of getting in foal again.

The growing foetus makes very few demands on the mare during the first eight months of its development. Although a tremendous amount of development is taking place, it is not actually growing fast enough to make any appreciable demands on the mare. Something like 80 per cent of foetal growth takes place in the last three months of gestation. In practical terms this means that, providing the mare is in good condition, she need only be fed a maintenance ration. Assuming that she conceives in April, grass keep should be adequate until September or October. Obviously this depends on the quantity and quality of the pasture, and a dry summer where keep is short would mean a revision of this plan. As the grass supply wanes, and providing that she is still in good condition, the mare should only need good quality hay until Christmas. Unless the mare is out on very heavy ground that poaches badly, is losing condition or the autumn is particularly wet, there is no reason why she should not stay out day and night until Christmas. Exercise is important to keep her physically fit and to facilitate foaling.

The mare must be wormed every four to six weeks and her feet and vaccinations kept up to date.

### Christmas to foaling

After Christmas the mare may need to come in at night, although there are no hard and fast rules and a part-bred mare may be happier out. A mare does not have to be stabled just because she is in foal. Now is the time to start introducing a concentrate feed unless, as with some native breeds, she is overweight.

During the last 90 days of pregnancy the foetus starts to grow rapidly and the mare's nutrient requirements increase. At the same time the foetus begins to occupy a greater proportion of the mare's abdomen; there is less room for her gut and consequently her appetite for bulk feed may fall. This must be made up by feeding a greater proportion of concentrate feed. The mare's nutrient requirements increase so that the developing foal's body tissue can be laid down, and this requires both energy and protein. The pregnant mare requires about 12 per cent protein in her diet overall; even good quality hay will only have a protein content of about 10 per cent, and this means that every kilogram of hay fed leads to a shortfall of protein of 2 per cent. In order to overcome this deficiency, the mare's concentrate feed should have a protein content of about 16 per cent.

The mare's feed should be gradually increased so that she maintains her condition: a 16.2 hh Thoroughbred mare may need as much as 6–7 kg (14–16 lb) of concentrate feed per day. It is equally important not to overfeed broodmares; it is a fallacy that only fat ponies are susceptible to laminitis – overfed barren and pregnant mares are equally at risk.

There is conflicting evidence about the effects of overfeeding and underfeeding in the last three months of pregnancy. Generally speaking, the fat mare should maintain, not lose, weight, and the thin mare should gain weight. Any imposed weight loss in obese brood mares should take place between the second and eighth month of pregnancy, and preferably before they are covered.

It is important that the diet is balanced in calcium and phosphorus: a lack or imbalance of either mineral will result in the mare using her own body resources, and in extreme cases will result in the foal being born weak.

**Table 8.2**    The minimum daily requirements of calcium and phosphorus.

| Age | Bodyweight (kg) | Calcium (g) | Phosphorus (g) | Limestone (g/day) | Dicalcium phosphate (g/day) |
|---|---|---|---|---|---|
| 3 months | 100 | 37 | 31 | 104 | 148 |
| 6 months | 200 | 33 | 27 | 92 | 108 |
| 12 months | 300 | 31 | 25 | 87 | 92 |
| Mature | 450 | 23 | 18 | 64 | 60 |
| Lactating | 500 | 33 | 23 | 92 | 108 |

## Feeding the pregnant mare (last 3 months)

**Table 8.3**    Ration for a pregnant mare.

| | |
|---|---|
| Digestible energy (MJ/kg of the diet) | 10.5 |
| Crude protein | 11% |
| Ratio of hay to concentrates | 65:35 |
| Calcium | 0.5% |
| Phosphorus | 0.35% |
| Hay of 8 MJ DE/kg | 8 kg (18 lb) |
| Concentrate of 11 MJ DE/kg | 4 kg (9 lb) |

} Ratio 1.5:1

The table shows a ration suitable for a 500 kg (1100 lb), 16 hh lightweight mare. She should receive 11 per cent crude protein in her ration and 10.5 MJ of digestible energy per kilogram of diet. If the hay is good quality this would be satisfied by a hay to concentrate ratio of 75:25, while if the hay was only medium quality the ratio would need to be 65:35. A suitable ration using average quality hay and a high protein stud cube would be 8 kg (18 lb) hay and 4 kg (9 lb) concentrate. Salt, limestone or dicalcium phosphate and cod liver oil should also be fed. As always this is only a guide; all horses are individuals and must be treated as such.

## Foaling

Some mares may naturally go off their feed as foaling approaches; do not panic, but lower her concentrate ration and let her eat as much good quality hay as she wants. In later-foaling mares the flush of spring grass will occur at about this time and may help reduce the problem of meconium retention in foals.

In the 24 hours before foaling, the mare should be fed good quality hay and low energy concentrates, e.g. horse and pony cubes with chaff, bran or sugar beet pulp. It is likely that the mare will go off her feed anyway. The first feed after foaling may usefully be the controversial bran mash, as this is appetising and easy to eat. The now-lactating mare will subsequently go onto a higher plane of nutrition.

## Feeding the barren or maiden mare

Providing that the barren mare is not too fat or too thin, a similar feeding regime to that of the mare in early pregnancy is suitable. A maintenance ration of good quality hay until Christmas should be adequate. At about Christmas the mare should be stabled at night, rugged and her stable light left on to give her 16 hours of light a day. She should be fed a concentrate feed once or twice a day. The idea is to persuade the mare's body systems that spring is on the way, and this starts her oestrous cycles earlier in the year than normal.

## Feeding the lactating broodmare

The fresh spring grass that should coincide with the mare foaling will meet all her requirements for energy, protein, calcium and phosphorus. Early-foaling mares being fed low-protein grass hay will need a stud diet with 16–17 per cent crude protein. The mare should not be overfed roughage as this may limit her capacity for concentrate; the hay to concentrate ratio will need to be higher than for pregnancy in order to meet the higher protein requirement at about 50:50.

A cereal mix can replace the stud cube but it must be supplemented with soyabean meal or another protein concentrate. A 550 kg mare on a grass hay and oat/barley diet would need 1.75 kg of soya a day to bring the protein level of the ration up to 12.5 per cent. It is very important to add salt and limestone to this cereal based ration as well as a mineral and vitamin mix.

## Feeding youngstock

Most farm animals have been selected for measurable traits such as growth rates and feed conversion efficiency, in other words how efficiently they convert food into meat, milk or eggs. This has led to a population of animals that grow in a fairly consistent way and it is possible to predict how feeding will affect the animals' growth rate and in turn how to produce rations that will help to attain maximum growth and to minimise growth-related problems. Horses have been selected for performance resulting in a diverse population; some grow more quickly than others, some are better 'doers' than others. As a result we do not really know the correct way to feed youngstock.

### Developmental Orthopaedic Disease

Growing horses may suffer various growth-related problems known as metabolic bone disease or developmental orthopaedic disease (DOD). The majority of these problems arise in the first year of the youngster's life. Unfortunately the role of nutrition in these problems is unclear, however, high energy and/or high protein diets inducing rapid growth have traditionally been associated with developmental orthopaedic diseases such as epiphysitis or angular limb deformities. As more work is done on DOD it would seem that other factors may be more important: nursing foals that are underfed, weanlings that lose weight after weaning and then overeat and grow too quickly, large, infrequent concentrate meals and mineral and vitamin imbalances may all be implicated in growth problems.

Frequently young horses are overfed; too much energy is provided in large infrequent meals of carbohydrate-rich concentrates. Horses are not designed to eat meals, they are trickle feeders and it has been suggested that large peaks in blood glucose occur after a horse has eaten a meal, this is followed by insulin surges as the horse attempts to regulate blood glucose levels. In turn there is a temporary decrease in thyroxine production by the thyroid gland. Thyroxine is involved in cartilage development and this sequence of events may be implicated in DOD.

## The foal

It is vital that the newborn foal receives adequate colostrum and suckles normally. Foals suckle very frequently, up to 100 times in 24 hours in the first week; small amounts of milk taken frequently are less likely to cause digestive upset. In the first few weeks of a foal's life the mare's milk provides all of its nutrition, thus the foal's growth rate will depend on how much milk the mare produces. The mare may produce 18–20 litres of fairly low quality milk per day (see Table 8.4).

Mare's milk may also be low in copper and iron, resulting in anaemia in very young foals which is not resolved until they begin to eat solid food.

By 10–21 days the foal should be nibbling hay, grass and concentrates and if the foal is being prepared for the show ring, for early performance

**Table 8.4**  Comparison of the milk composition of domestic animals.

|      | % water | % protein | % fat | % sugar | % minerals |
|------|---------|-----------|-------|---------|------------|
| Mare | 89.5    | 2.5       | 1.5   | 6.0     | 0.5        |
| Cow  | 87.0    | 3.5       | 3.8   | 5.0     | 0.7        |
| Ewe  | 83.0    | 5.4       | 6.5   | 4.3     | 1.0        |

like flat racing, or if the mare is short of milk, then the foal should be creep fed. Creep feeding is the method of giving the foal a special concentrate feed that is not available to its mother, so that the foal's growth is accelerated and the digestive tract is developed so that weaning is not so traumatic. A creep feed based on skimmed milk (18% crude protein) can be used from two weeks onwards. The amount of creep feed that the foal will require in the first few weeks depends largely on the mare's milk yield. From 10–14 weeks the feed should be gradually changed to a growing foal diet or stud cube (14–16% crude protein). Milk pellets should not really be fed prior to weaning as the foal's gut must be taught to digest other nutrients.

Foals that are growing well do not need a creep until about eight weeks before weaning. The idea is to:

- compensate for the mare's falling milk yield
- compensate for the decline in pasture quality
- accustom the foal's gut to concentrates.

The creep feed eaten will probably be about 0.5–0.75 kg per 100 kg bodyweight. To put this in perspective, a foal likely to weigh 550 kg at maturity (a 16 hh middleweight), will weigh approximately 150–200 kg at weaning and will be eating 1–1.5 kg of concentrate feed. A useful rule of thumb is to provide 450 g creep feed per day for each month of age.

Foals can suffer from growth related problems such as epiphysitis and contracted tendons. If these problems arise then both the mare's and the foal's concentrate feed should be cut out for three to four weeks. This restriction will not affect the foal's mature weight if it is carefully regulated. Foals that are born high on their toes should be turned out to grass as soon as possible and not allowed to grow too quickly.

## Weanlings

Naturally the foal should be weaned about a month before the mare's next foal is due, by this time the youngster should be very independent and the procedure not traumatic. However, most studs wean foals at about six months of age, giving the mare a respite from lactation during the winter months and facilitating youngstock management. At this age weaning is stressful and foals that are separated from their mothers can become very distressed. Careful management can reduce the stress of weaning and it is important that the foals are adapted to solid feed. Foals that do not eat enough immediately after weaning may lose weight while greedy foals may eat too much. Both over and under feeding alters growth rates and may result in the foal developing bone abnormalities.

Weaning often takes place in September or October, just as the grass quality is declining, this means that grass will provide few nutrients for the weanling. The young horse must be accustomed to a high quality concentrate feed containing the nutrients needed for optimum growth during this critical period. Feeding good quality roughage is also important and moderate hay can be supplemented with alfalfa.

Weanlings may be yarded during their first winter, this allows them plenty of room for exercise while being kept warm and sheltered. However, a watch must be kept for bullying at feed time. Some studs feed a complete ration consisting of an ad lib supply of chopped forage and concentrate, if it is not practical to feed a complete ration it is useful to feed a reputable stud cube, designed for young growing horses, along with good quality hay during the winter. It is unlikely that a weanling would need more than 3.5 kg of concentrates if allowed as much hay as it wanted. Unless the weanling is being prepared for sale or show, it should be possible to feel a rib with no appreciable layer of fat. The growing horse should always have its diet supplemented with calcium and phosphorus to ensure good bone growth.

### Yearlings

#### Energy

Low energy levels reduce growth rates while too much energy causes obesity, puts a strain on the horse's limbs and may contribute to DOD. The weanling needs about 13 MJ DE/kg of diet and the yearling about 12 MJ DE/kg. As even good quality roughages may only contain about 8–9 MJ DE/kg the young horse needs to eat more concentrate than roughage, usually a ratio of 70 per cent concentrate to 30 per cent roughage for the weanling and 55 per cent concentrate and 45 per cent hay for the yearling (Table 8.7). If poor quality roughage is used either the amount of concentrate fed must be increased or a higher energy concentrate used. As the growth rate of the yearling slows down so the energy requirement falls until the horse is mature. As this happens the roughage component of the ration becomes more important (Table 8.5) and eventually the mature horse can maintain its body weight on roughage alone. In practical terms, if a stud compound containing 11 MJ DE/kg and 16 per cent crude protein is used to feed a Thoroughbred-type horse expected to make 16 hh at maturity, a weanling would receive 2 kg of hay and 4 kg of concentrate while a yearling would be fed 3.5 kg of hay and 4 kg of stud compound. Obviously this is only a guideline and the condition of the youngster must be monitored and the feeding adjusted accordingly.

**Table 8.5**  Ratio of forage to concentrate.

|  | Age (months) | Concentrate | Hay |
|---|---|---|---|
| Weanling | 6 | 70 | 30 |
| Yearling | 12 | 60 | 40 |
| Yearling | 18 | 45 | 55 |
| Two-year-old | 24 | 35 | 65 |

## Protein

Protein is needed for the growth and development of all tissues (Table 8.6) and it is important to remember that the quality of the protein is as important as the quantity. An adequate supply of indispensable amino acids is vital for correct growth and development with the levels of lysine being particularly important. Lysine is deficient in many conventional feedstuffs and a stud ration based on straights can be improved by the addition of soyabean meal which is a good source of high quality protein. Lysine is also low in poor quality roughage.

**Table 8.6**  Protein requirements of youngstock.

|  | Age (months) | Crude protein (%) |
|---|---|---|
| Weanling | 6 | 16 |
| Yearling | 12 | 13.5 |
| Yearling | 18 | 11.5 |
| Two-year-old | 24 | 10 |

*Minerals and vitamins*

Calcium, phosphorus, copper, magnesium and zinc are all important for growth and development and are likely to be deficient in a traditional ration so should be supplied by using a suitable supplement. A stud compound should contain adequate amounts of micronutrients but the levels of calcium and phosphorus may be marginal and need 'topping up' with dicalcium phosphate or another suitable source.

Giving young horses a good start is the first step on the road which will help them realise their full athletic potential; however, our limited knowledge of youngstock nutrition can make it difficult for the owner to decide on the correct type and amounts of feed to give. As always there are no hard and fast rules but bear in mind the following points:

- Feed the best quality hay you can afford.
- If the hay is not high quality substitute some hay by dried chopped alfalfa. Alfalfa is a high fibre source of protein, calcium and beta-carotene (vitamin A precursor).
- Alternatively adjust the ratio of forage to concentrate to provide adequate nutrients.
- Supplement an oat-based ration with soyabean meal and a suitable mineral and vitamin supplement *or* use a specially formulated compound feed, and feed as specified by the manufacturer.
- Keep an eye on condition and rate of growth.
- Do not rely on pasture, its nutrient value is highly variable in terms of quality and quantity.
- Feed adequate calcium and phosphorus.

## Feeding the stallion

Out of the breeding season, the stallion in good condition should maintain his condition on good quality hay and horse and pony cubes. This plane of nutrition should be gradually increased after Christmas, as exercise is introduced to fitten him for the covering season. During the covering season stallions may become difficult to feed, refusing to eat and losing condition. They should be fed a stud cube or equivalent concentrate mix and good quality hay at the rate of 0.75–1.5 kg per 100 kg bodyweight, i.e. 3.75–7.5 kg for a 16.2 hh Thoroughbred stallion of 500 kg. Generally speaking, the stallion should be fed as if he is doing moderately hard work, with good quality palatable feed and a general mineral and vitamin supplement. Whilst a deficiency of vitamin E has been implicated in fertility problems, feeding extra vitamin E does not guarantee extra fertility.

## Feeding the orphan foal

If a foster mother cannot be found for an orphan foal it may have to be hand-reared; a feeding bottle can be made by fitting a clean soft-drink bottle with a lamb teat. The foal should be taught to drink milk from a bucket as soon as possible: allowing the foal to lick milk off the fingers and then immersing the fingers in the bucket will encourage the foal to follow the finger and discover the milk. It must never be forced to put its head in the bucket.

If the foal is premature or lacks a normal suck reflex, it must be fed through a stomach tube until it has learned to suckle. A soft rubber tube is passed into the foal's nostril, down its throat and into its stomach. Milk is then slowly poured into a funnel attached to the tube. The foal's nostril should be greased and when the tube reaches the back of its throat the foal should swallow so that the tube passes down the gullet, not into the lungs. The handler must listen to the end of the tube before putting any milk down the tube. If the tube is in the lungs a characteristic noise will be heard and the tube should be slowly withdrawn. A vet must show you how to use the stomach tube correctly.

A reputable mare's milk replacer, made up as directed, should be used; cow's milk is too rich but goat's milk can be used. During the first two weeks, normal healthy foals should be fed every two hours and during the second two weeks they should be fed every four hours. They should then be fed four times a day until weaning. The amount and frequency of feeds needed will vary according to the size, age and state of health of the individual foal, but initially foals should be fed about a quarter of a pint (142 ml) at each feed. Each week the amount fed should be increased to the maximum that the foal will eat without scouring. Scouring without fever or any other signs of illness may indicate that the foal is being overfed and its diet should be adjusted accordingly.

The orphan foal should be introduced to solid feed as quickly as possible; this will encourage gut development and allow the foal to be weaned from the bucket earlier. Pellets containing milk or milk replacer pellets can be added to the bucket of milk replacer, which will encourage the foal to eat them. The pellets should contain at least 16–18 per cent high quality protein, and have a high energy content and adequate levels of minerals and vitamins, particularly calcium and phosphorus.

The hand-reared orphan foal should be weaned from milk replacers when possible; early weaning will save labour costs and allow the foal to lead a more normal life. The foal must look well and be adequately creep fed; the milk ration should be gradually reduced and creep feeding continued for another three months.

## General guidelines for feeding stud stock

- Feed good quality forage.
- If forage is not good quality make good the shortfall by feeding extra concentrates or alfalfa.
- Do not rely solely on pasture; its quality can vary dramatically depending on time of year, sward quality and soil nutrition. Compensate for pasture inadequacy with concentrates.
- Constantly check condition and growth rates to avoid poor conformation and developmental orthopaedic disease.
- Feed adequate calcium and phosphorus in the correct ratio and quantity.
- Only use one good general mineral, vitamin and amino acid supplement. Except in specific cases the use of more than one supplement may imbalance the ration further, as they may not complement each other.

## Feeding for performance

Overfeeding or underfeeding will impair a horse's performance; a good trainer is one who can balance the horse's work and feed to produce an athlete ready to give his best. Generalisations are always a mistake, and it is just as difficult to compare the feeding of a horse training for Badminton to that of a five-year old in its first season's eventing as it is to compare the Golden Horseshoe horse and one competing in Pleasure Rides. However a few general guidelines are the same for all horses, regardless of the competitive goal:

- Once a horse is receiving his full ration of concentrates he should be given at least three feeds a day. If the horse is not eating up, give a late night feed, so that he is getting the same weight of feed but in four smaller feeds.

**Table 8.7**  Summary of feeding stud stock.

| Type of horse | DE (MJ DE/kg) | Ratio of concentrate to hay | | Crude protein (%) | Ca (%) | P (%) | Vitamin A (iu/kg) | Ration | | | |
| | | Good hay (10 MJ De/kg) | Medium hay (8 MJ DE/kg) | | | | | Hay | | Cube* | |
| | | | | | | | | (kg) | (lb) | (kg) | (lb) |
| --- | --- | --- | --- | --- | --- | --- | --- | --- | --- | --- | --- |
| Breeding stallion | 12 | 50:50 | 45:55 | 10 | 0.45 | 0.35 | 2450 | 7 | 15 | 5 | 11 |
| Pregnant mare (last 3 months) | 10.5 | 25:75 | 35:65 | 10 | 0.5 | 0.35 | 3400 | 7.5 | 16.5 | 4.5 | 10 |
| Lactating mare (first 3 months) | 12 | 45:55 | 55:45 | 12.5 | 0.5 | 0.35 | 2800 | 5 | 11 | 7 | 15 |
| Lactating mare (second 3 months) | 11 | 30:70 | 40:60 | 11 | 0.45 | 0.3 | 2450 | 7.5 | 16.5 | 5 | 11 |
| Weanling | 13 | 65:35 | 70:30 | 16 | 0.85 | 0.6 | 2000 | 2 | 4.5 | 4 | 9 |
| Yearling | 12 | 45:55 | 50:50 | 13.5 | 0.55 | 0.4 | 2000 | 3.5 | 8 | 3.5 | 8 |
| Two-year-old | 11 | 30:70 | 40:60 | 10 | 0.45 | 0.35 | 2000 | 5 | 11 | 2.5 | 5.5 |

NB: the compound contains 11 MJ DE/kg and 16% crude protein. Salt, limestone or dicalcium phosphate and codliver oil should be fed to satisfy the requirement for calcium, phosphorus and vitamin A.
The quality and quantity of grazing available will alter the amounts fed.

- If the horse is not getting out to grass he should have his hay ration divided into three, with the largest amount being given at night. It is not good for the horse to go for long periods of time without food in his gut; if he is given his hay at 5 pm and not fed until 8 am the following morning, he may well go over 12 hours with no food, so try to make the evening hay ration as large as possible.
- The horse should have a salt lick in the manger; this will help to stop him bolting his feed and provide him with a minimum amount of salt. Many horses in hard work that are sweating heavily will not get enough salt from this lick. As soon as your horse starts to do any fast work he should be given 60 g (2 oz) of salt in his evening feed.
- Fresh clean water should be available at all times; drinkers and buckets must be regularly scrubbed out.
- The concentrate feed intake must always be severely restricted if the horse has to be laid off work. On a rest day the concentrate ration should be halved and the hay increased. If your horse goes out in the field on his day off and is not receiving more than 5 kg (11 lb) of hard feed, you may get away with keeping the feed level the same, but do take care.

## Eventing

The event horse has to be fit enough to gallop and jump at speed, and yet disciplined enough to perform dressage and show jumping. This has led to many event riders trying to keep their horses happy mentally and physically by feeding as few concentrates as possible and turning their horses out in the field every day. The three-day event horse may have a very rigorous training programme and yet only compete in a few events on the run up to the main competition before being turned away, while the lower level horse may compete once a week throughout the long event season. These horses have widely differing feed requirements.

Many riders worry about the amount their horse eats during a two or three day event, but as long as the horse is eating its hay and drinking normally, there is no need to worry unduly. The horse has enough energy stored in its liver and muscles to see it through three days of competition. Prior to the event do not be tempted to change the horse's ration. Some people reduce or cut out the sugar beet pulp before the event, while others would only reduce or omit the beet pulp on the morning of cross-country day. If the horse frets away from home, reduce the quantity of concentrate food and use high energy palatable ingredients such as milk pellets and flaked maize. Generally speaking though it is better not to fiddle with the horse's feed too much: you may just cause problems.

A three-day event horse should have a concentrate feed no less than four hours before the start time of Phase A. If he is competing in the afternoon he could also have a small haynet. If the horse has had free access to fresh water there is no reason why he should have his water bucket taken away before he competes – why should he suddenly decide to have a huge drink?

A novice event horse could munch on a haynet while being plaited on the morning of his competition; if he has early times he should not receive any bulk while travelling until after his cross-country. If his cross-country time is late he could have a small haynet while travelling. Depending on your times, he may be able to have a concentrate feed between the dressage and the show jumping, providing that there is at least two hours digestion time. He should be offered water frequently throughout the day and allowed to wash his mouth out between the show jumping and the cross-country, even if they are very close together.

The fluid and electrolyte balance is very important, and the horse must be watched for signs of dehydration. If a pinch of skin on the neck or shoulder lingers after it has been released, and the horse has a gaunt tucked-in appearance, it may well be dehydrated – this really can limit the next day's performance severely. Ensure that the horse drinks and provide electrolytes in the food or water.

Colic can be a problem after severe exertion, and the intestines must be kept moving. Once the horse is cool and his thirst has been quenched he may appreciate a small bran mash, with his normal feed later on. Tired horses are easily over-faced by a large feed, but dividing the normal feed in two, and feeding it at intervals, may overcome this.

After the competition the horse's appetite will tell you how tired he has been. Until he is eating up normally, he has not really recovered from his exertions and should be allowed plenty of rest. Hacks and grazing in hand will help the horse relax and recover.

## Endurance and long distance horses

Horses competing in long distance rides have to learn to make effective use of body fat reserves as a source of energy and as a way of conserving the precious limited glucose reserves. Once all the glucose stores have been used up, the horse will become fatigued. Horses fed corn oil have been shown to digest it very efficiently, and high levels of dietary fat slow down the drop in blood glucose during endurance work. It would seem that a high fat diet, containing 8–12 per cent total fat, may stimulate the body to use it as an energy source, thus conserving glucose and allowing the horse to work longer before it becomes fatigued.

In practical terms providing 8–12 per cent fat in the diet means feeding 1–1.5 litres (2–3 pints) of oil a day. This is a very high level and although I have successfully fed 0.5 litres (1 pint) a day, more work needs to be done before this can be recommended. Half a litre of oil is equivalent in energy terms to feeding 18 MJ DE per day and means that you can drop your concentrate ration by 1.5 kg (3.5 lb) of oats per day. This is useful if you have a horse that is difficult to keep in condition or which tends to get very excitable on a high concentrate diet. Oil is digested in the small intestine, unlike cereals, where starch may pass to the large intestine to be fermented by the bacteria as outlined earlier. Substituting oil for some of the cereal part of a ration may stop the horse being as 'hot'.

The provision of water for the endurance horse is vitally important, and he should be accustomed to drinking during the ride whenever possible; giving water little and often prevents dehydration without causing problems. Electrolytes are very important to endurance horses; they can be given in a horse's feed for a day or two prior to the ride, and during the ride in water and sugar beet liquid. Sometimes they are given by syringing concentrated electrolyte solution into the horse's mouth during a ride, but this must never be done before the horse has started to drink well, or the strong salt solution in the horse's stomach will cause fluid to be drawn into the stomach from the tissues, to dilute the solution. This will in fact cause dehydration, so remember that over-use or incorrect use of electrolytes can be harmful.

## Showjumping and dressage

Showjumpers and dressage horses are both trained to perform tests of obedience and accuracy, which require considerable power at more advanced levels. They do not perform fast work or endurance work and do not need to be as lean as the endurance horse or eventer. Frequently they are strongly muscled and carry quite a lot of condition. By contrast both dressage horses and showjumpers may compete very frequently with a long competition season. The skill in feeding these horses is to keep their condition and to keep them mentally fresh without over or under-feeding them. It is equally important to achieve the correct overall energy content of the diet in these horses as it is in racehorses.

# Racing

The two-year-old sprinting Thoroughbred is a very different creature to the Grand National horse. The way in which they are trained develops the muscle metabolism in different ways. The sprinter produces the energy for muscle contraction by the breakdown of glucose in the absence of oxygen – anaerobic respiration. The stayer produces much of the energy needed by burning up glucose in the presence of oxygen – aerobic respiration. Both have a very high energy requirement and the young horse will also have a high protein requirement; however overfeeding has been shown to depress performance.

In many racing yards horses are fed along traditional lines with a ration based on oats and grass hay. As we have seen, the nutrient composition of both these can be very variable, particularly in their protein content, so it is wise to check:

- The protein content of hay and any cereals fed.
- The lysine content of hay and any cereals fed to young working horses.
- That both the calcium:phosphorus ratio and the actual calcium intake are correct.
- That adequate salt is provided, especially in hot weather.
- That any supplement used provides correct levels of micronutrients, especially folic acid and possibly other water-soluble vitamins.
- That vitamins A and D are not overfed.
- Supplements are not mixed as they may not complement one another.

# Feeding on journeys

One of the major problems horses experience when travelling long distances is dehydration. It is very important to offer the horse water at frequent intervals. If the horse is sweating it is wise to include some electrolytes. Some horses are more fussy about water than they are about food, so take water from home in a couple of containers, so that the taste of unfamiliar water will not put the horse off drinking. If you have a real problem then try adding a little molasses to the water at home so that you can do the same at your destination and disguise the different taste. Fortunately most horses will drink when they are thirsty, no matter what it tastes like.

The horse will spend a long time standing still during the journey, and you do not want his legs to fill or for him to experience any other

**Table 8.8**  Rations for 15.2–16 hh, 500 kg horse at different work levels.

| Work level | Digestible energy required (MJ/kg) | Crude protein required (%) | Ratio of hay to concentrates | Ration | | | | Comments |
|---|---|---|---|---|---|---|---|---|
| | | | | Hay (8 MJ DE/kg) | | Concentrate | | |
| | | | | (kg) | (lb) | (kg) | (lb) | |
| Maintenance | 9 | 7.5 | 90:10 | 9.5 | 21 | 1 | 2 | Horse and pony cubes (10 MJ DE/kg) |
| Light (getting fit) | 9.5 | 8 | 80:20 | 8.5 | 19 | 2 | 4.5 | As above |
| Light to medium (Novice horse trials) | 10 | 8.5 | 70:30 | 7.5 | 16 | 3.5 | 8 | Event cubes (11 MJ DE/kg) |
| Medium (Intermediate horse trials) | 11 | 9 | 60:40 | 6.5 | 14 | 5 | 11 | As above |
| Hard (Advanced horse trials) | 12 | 9.5 | 40:60 | 5.5 | 12 | 6.5 | 14 | Racehorse cubes (14 MJ DE/kg) or oats plus protein concentrate |
| Fast (Racing) | 13.5 | 10–11 | 30:70 | 3.5 | 7.5 | 8.5 | 18 | As above |

metabolic upsets, so this means the concentrate ration must be cut down. On the other hand you do not want the fit horse to lose condition. This dilemma is best solved by allowing the horse plenty of good quality hay during the journey, so that his gut is kept moving and partially-full the whole time; this will reduce the risk of colic. The concentrate feeds could be small and easily digested and given at regular intervals. It may be useful to give the horse a bran mash the evening before the journey and only hay or a very small feed, including bran, the morning before setting off.

The rules of rationing have been used to produce the tables in Chapter 5 which are designed to act as a guideline for preparing rations for different types of horses.

## Feeding the obese horse

This problem is frequently encountered and much neglected by the 'experts', who tend to concentrate their efforts on racehorses and the like. People with fat youngsters are often advised to wait until they start to exercise them to get rid of the young horse's fat. This is not really satis-factory; if spring is rapidly approaching, the last thing anyone wants is a laminitic youngster. Riding him while he is overweight will also put enormous strain on his limbs, which have not yet stopped growing. So his weight must be gradually reduced before the flush of spring grass; he can then be broken or rebacked and the weight loss accelerated as he gets fitter. However, just like humans, this will be a slow process; in fact (within reason) the longer it takes to get the weight off the more likely it is to stay off.

- Reduce the amount of hay fed in the field during the day.
- Give a very small concentrate feed to provide the necessary minerals and vitamins; add some limestone to his feed, particularly if he is going to have his hay ration cut.
- If he is in at night try turning him out all the time with a small amount of hay.
- If he is out at night then do not feed him any hay in the evening. He can wander round the field all night thus exercising himself and dieting himself at the same time.
- If you already do all these things and they do not work then he is going to have to be brought in and fed a restricted diet.
- There is every chance that he is going to feel quite hungry and he may

become bad-tempered. Try to ignore this and carry on as normal; it will be worth it in the long run.

Once the horse has lost weight he must not get fat again; many horses will never be able to have as much food as they want.

## Feeding the show horse

In order to be successful in the show-ring young horses need more than good conformation; they must be very well grown and be well covered and round to the point of nearly being fat. To do the early shows requires a lot of preparation. The horse must be stabled at night and well rugged up for Christmas; this will help the horse change its coat early and stop it using up food to keep warm.

### Yearlings

The young show horse needs a high energy and protein ration that is going to help it put on condition quickly, but the ration must be balanced in minerals and vitamins so that it does not get any problems associated with rapid growth, such as epiphysitis. Exercise is helpful, walking in hand for 30 minutes a day; this will teach manners and help develop the correct muscles.

Feed must be good quality: if the hay is not up to scratch, substitute some haylage or alfalfa chaff; the horse does not want to be filled up with food of low nutrient quality. Yearlings have a high protein requirement because they are still growing; provide this protein as a yearling cube, a balancer cube to be fed with cereals, or by feeding extracted soyabean meal. Extra energy can be given as vegetable cooking oil: start off with a tablespoon a day and gradually work up to 300 ml (a mugful) a day. This is equivalent to about 1 kg (2 lb) of oats and will also do wonders for the coat. Minerals and vitamins must also be added if not using a cube; a good quality all round supplement with adequate levels of lysine is advisable. Limestone, about 80 g per day, must also be added and there should be a salt lick in the manger.

Yearlings may benefit from probiotics, to help the gut cope with this rich diet. Keep a close watch on the joints and if they become warm and filled, cut the concentrates immediately, feeding only hay until they return to normal. If the horse gets very above itself, try more exercise, longer in the field or a change of diet.

A suggested ration for a yearling is:

| | |
|---|---|
| Hay | 3.5 kg (7 lb) |
| Yearling cubes | 3.5 kg (7 lb)* |
| Alfalfa chaff | 0.5 kg (1 lb) |
| Vegetable oil | 300 ml |
| Limestone | 80 g |
| Sugar beet pulp | 0.5 kg (1 lb) (dry weight) |

*An alternative to the yearling cubes would be 3 kg (6 lb) micronised barley + 0.5 kg (1 lb) extracted soyabean meal + 0.5 kg (1 lb) grass/alfalfa cubes + supplement.

## Feeding horses at grass

Hayracks must be a safe design and moved regularly to prevent poaching. The design often used for cattle with a feeding trough underneath is not suitable: it allows seeds to drop in the horse's eyes and has sharp corners on which a horse can hurt itself (Fig. 8.1). Some of the round cattle feeders are useful but must be of a type where a horse cannot hit its head or become trapped. The rack must be heavy enough not to be easily pushed over when empty. Racks should be placed in a well-drained spot, away from the fence, with good clearance all round.

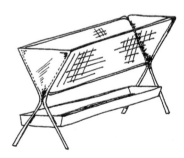

**Fig. 8.1** Hay rack and feeder not suitable for horses.

Haynets must be tied securely to a solid fencepost or tree, so that they will hang just over the top of the horse's leg when empty: otherwise the horse may get its feet tangled in them. Obviously this is tricky if you are feeding groups of horses as they will be different sizes. In this case hay is best fed on the floor – wastage is better than an accident. One more haynet or heap of hay should be put out than there are horses, and they should be well spaced out so that kicking and bullying is minimised.

Concentrate feeding should be supervised, as it is a time when horses can be very aggressive and accidents can happen. Always feed all the horses at the same time, or take out the horse to be fed and feed it out of sight of the others. There are a variety of buckets and troughs which can be hung over a post and rail fence, although these can be knocked off and spill. Non-spill feeders for feeding from the ground can be purchased or a bucket can be dropped into a close-fitting tyre.

# Chapter 9
# The Added Extras

## Supplements

Every horsey magazine is full of adverts for feed supplements, each one claiming to be the best for your horse – making it stay healthy, jump higher or run faster. How is the horse owner to decide which supplement to use and when?

It is important to realise that a supplement is not a recipe for success – it can only work if it corrects an imbalance or deficiency in the horse's diet. So before choosing a supplement ask yourself if your horse really needs one; ask the advice of an independent equine nutritionist or a vet who has a thorough knowledge of horse nutrition. Horses likely to require a supplement are stabled performance horses, growing youngsters, broodmares in late pregnancy and early lactation, old horses and those receiving poor quality hay, especially in winter. A traditional mixture of corn and hay provides inadequate amounts of calcium for young horses and lactating mares; they will need a supplement. Ideally every horse would have its requirements matched to the nutrient specification of the feeds available, and a specially mixed supplement designed to balance that ration, but this is not an option for most horse owners. Some race-horse trainers have their hay analysed for protein and energy and let the feed compounder provide them with an appropriate cube or coarse mix which is then balanced with a compatible supplement.

There may be marked regional variations in the minerals in the soil, which can affect the grazing horse and horses eating hay or grain grown on that land. Ask your vet or local agricultural advisory service (ADAS): they should be able to tell you if there are any special requirements for your area.

Supplements are substances added to the horse's diet to balance it by filling in deficiencies of certain nutrients, most often minerals, vitamins and amino acids. An additive is something which is added to an already balanced ration, for example probiotics and enzymes; these may have an indirect effect on the horse's health but they are not fed for their nutritional value.

Supplements can vary in their complexity: one of the most simple supplements fed to horses is salt (sodium chloride), while at the other end of the scale there are broad spectrum supplements containing many nutrients. Broad spectrum supplements are formulated on the basis of the average horse being fed an average ration, making up for likely deficiencies; some simple supplements cater for specific problems, e.g. biotin for hoof growth.

The ingredients within a supplement may be natural or synthetic: many vitamins can be manufactured and are often more active than the natural vitamin source. This means that the sources of nutrients must be considered when comparing supplements. Many brands contain a mixture of synthetic and natural nutrient sources.

## Guidelines for feeding supplements

(1) Never mix or overdose supplements, unless recommended to do so by your vet or nutritionist. Just because 25 g of supplement is required does not mean to say that 50 g is going to be twice as good – you may be creating an imbalance as bad as the one you are trying to correct. The only things that you will probably have to add are salt and calcium.

(2) Remember that compound feeds are already supplemented; if you are feeding your horse the maximum amount of cubes recommended by the manufacturers he should not need another supplement. If you are feeding a cube at half the recommended level, feed a suitable supplement at half dose. If your horse looks well and is performing well, why waste money?

(3) Split the supplement between all the feeds; do not give it all in the evening feed as we all tend to do. The rules of feeding say make any changes gradually and if the horse's evening feed is different from the rest due to the supplements, nutrients will be wasted.

(4) If you are feeding a hot feed like a mash, wait for it to cool down before adding the supplement, otherwise nutrients may be denatured. If you feed a bran mash be sure to add some extra calcium to compensate for the low calcium level in bran.

(5) Like any new feed, introduce supplements gradually, taking about a week to build up to the full dose.

(6) Mix the supplement thoroughly into the feed, taking particular care if

you are mixing one big feed for a group of horses – one might end up with all the supplement.

### Supplement format

Supplements come in various forms: liquids, powders, meals or pellets.

#### Liquids

These are usually palatable sweet syrups. They help keep the dust down but can be difficult to mix – sticking everywhere. They are usually dispensed in a measured dose by a pump, which is useful on a large yard where the difference between a level scoop and a heaped scoop of powdered supplement could soon add up.

#### Powder

Not very practical for outdoor use as it can blow away. Try putting the supplement on the feed and then putting soaked sugar beet pulp on top so that when you mix the feed the supplement does not blow away or just stick to the edge of the feed bucket.

#### Meal

This is usually a powdered supplement that has been premixed onto bran or wheatfeed, making it easier to mix into the feed. Settling can occur, so tip the tub up and give it a good shake every so often.

#### Pellets

These are usually palatable and are useful if the horse is only having a tiny feed.

#### Injections

Certain supplements, for example vitamin $B_{12}$, may be given under veterinary supervision for specific reasons. It is probably not good practice to give routine vitamin shots; proper balanced nutrition should make this unnecessary. If the horse's metabolism is suddenly exposed to very high doses of a nutrient they will not be utilised efficiently; a horse will best use what its metabolism is 'trained' to deal with.

## What to look for in a supplement

### Salt

Whatever diet you are feeding you will need to add salt. The performance horse should have at least 40 g per day of common salt added to his feeds, with a salt lick in his manger for insurance. Horses and ponies that are not working so hard could rely on a salt lick either in their manger or out in the field. Grazing horses that eat soil and bark are almost certainly seeking salt.

### Calcium

On a grass hay/cereal diet you will need to add calcium; 25–30 g per day of limestone flour is a minimum requirement. Most broad spectrum supplements will contain some calcium and phosphorus but not enough to balance the ration. The manufacturer does not know what you are going to feed, and the calcium and phosphorus requirements will vary depending on the horse's diet, age and reproductive status.

### Vitamins and minerals

A stabled horse is likely to require vitamins A, D and E, plus folic acid. A selection of B vitamins may be necessary for performance horses receiving more than 50 per cent of their diet as concentrates. Of all the trace elements, inadequate intakes of copper, selenium, manganese, iodine and zinc are most frequently detected and should be included in a supplement. The form of mineral can affect its availability to the horse as well as how it will interact with other nutrients; for instance iron affects the uptake of vitamin E. Unless you are feeding a high quality protein look out for lysine and methionine in your supplement.

## Buying supplements

(1) Supplements do not keep for ever, so buy from a supplier with a rapid turnover and always check the 'sell by' date. The tub should not have been stored by a heater, in direct sunlight or in the damp – all these factors will cause vitamins to deteriorate more rapidly.

(2) Look for a pack that is easy to reseal; if the tub is left open to the air it will deteriorate.

(3) Detailed but clear feeding instructions are essential. A flat dose rate cannot possibly suit all horses at all times. It is useful to have instructions that tell you how much to feed per 100 kg of bodyweight to horses performing different levels of work, or at different ages and reproductive states.

(4) Always read the instructions carefully and use the scoop provided. Remember that a heaped scoop can weigh half as much again as a level scoop.

## Electrolytes

During work the horse's muscles produce heat. This heat has to be lost from the body to prevent heatstroke, and the most efficient heat-loss mechanism is sweating. Sweating involves the evaporation of fluid (containing salts) from the surface of the horse's skin, taking with it excess heat. The horse may lose 10–12 litres (2 gallons) of sweat an hour in prolonged exercise. If forced to continue the horse will become dehydrated, exhausted and unable to continue further.

The salts or electrolytes lost in horse sweat are principally sodium and chloride, with lesser amounts of potassium, calcium and magnesium. Supplements of electrolytes are designed partially to replenish these losses and to help the horse recover from its exertions more swiftly. It is often necessary to give electrolytes before the horse will drink, if it has become very dehydrated.

## Herbs – a natural alternative

Natural remedies are becoming increasingly popular amongst horse owners as they become aware of the value of these treatments over and above the synthetic alternatives. Herbal treatments can be used to support the horse's health and his ability to cope with demanding activities without infringing any of the rules and regulations governing competitions.

### What are herbs?

Herbs are slow-growing, deep-rooted plants containing a wide range of nutrients. They are abundant in old-fashioned permanent pasture but as modern agriculture has become more intensive herbs have become considered as weeds and eliminated.

Feeding herbs is said to help prevent disease and other health problems occurring, although you must remember they cannot work miracles and a lot will depend on the severity of the disease and the age and health of the individual horse. The effects of feeding herbs are cumulative and act slowly; this is a considerable advantage because it gives the body time to adjust and respond, preventing stressful imbalances occurring. The benefits creep up on you. Feeding herbs to excess will not make them work better or quicker and may well be harmful in the long run.

## The principles of herbal treatment

The principle of herbal treatments is that the whole body is affected; they balance the body's systems – circulatory, respiratory, lymphatic, digestive, muscular, skeletal, immune, reproductive, urinary and glandular systems will all benefit. Any upset of the body's ability to keep its internal environment stable (known as homeostasis) will cause health problems. The more we ask of the horse in terms of performance and travel, combined with an artificial diet, the more we stress him. His chances of full athletic function and resistance to bacterial and viral infection will depend on his body's ability to adjust the homeostatic balance. The aim of the traditional herbalist is to piece together all the signs and symptoms shown by the patient and obtain an overall view of the body's disharmony, from which a herbal prescription can logically follow. This is obviously far more tricky for the veterinary herbalist and as always the observant horse owner will be a great help.

As the demands of the horse's systems increase, so does its demand for nutrients. There may even be a need for nutrients that have not yet been identified. Consequently herbs are beneficial because they contain a vast number of nutrients and chemicals in a balanced form.

Herbs may be given as a medicine in a concentrated form, prescribed by a vet specialising in herbal medicine. Many vets are becoming more interested in these types of alternative medicines – it is worth talking to your local vet. Many recognised active ingredients for medicines are extracted from herbs. This goes against the principles of herbalism; herbalists suggest that the plant – including seeds, root and bark – is a balanced entity and extracting one component will not produce the best results. The whole plant should be used so that the parts work together.

## The effects of a modern diet

Think of what we do to our horses' digestive systems: we give them additives, supplements and large quantities of highly processed concentrate feeds at times that fit in with our schedule. Add to this medications, wormers, antibiotics, steroids and painkillers and you can see that their diet is vastly different from their natural grazing habit. A more natural, high fibre diet is digested in the horse's hind gut with the aid of naturally occurring micro-organisms – this takes time and occupies a large volume. These 'good' bacteria are easily destroyed by digestive disturbances, further upsetting gut function. The highly concentrated diet of the performance horse is digested more quickly and earlier in the digestive system, in an unnatural process which may produce substances which adversely affect the gut bacteria. Many herbs support digestive function.

## The action and use of herbs

You can feed herbs as part of your horse's diet to act as a general support, or you can feed specific herbs to support a specific system.

Herbs can be grown easily and fed fresh or dried for winter use. Herbal supplements can be purchased and given in the feed – this is easier for many people as a couple of measures may be the equivalent of pounds of fresh material. Herbs can also be used to treat external problems and can act as healing agents and poultices.

**Table 9.1**   The action of herbs.

| | |
|---|---|
| Demulcents | Rich in mucilage. Soothe and protect inflamed and irritated tissue. |
| Bitters | Tone and normalise the digestive process and relieve absorption difficulties. |
| Anthelmintics | Work against parasitic worms. |
| Carminatives | Support natural movement of the intestines and passage of food through gut. |
| Antimicrobials | Support digestion during illness. |
| Vulneries | Promote healing of minor cuts and abrasions. |
| Alternatives | Correct blood pollution. |
| Antimicrobials | Cleanse the whole body. |

## Commonly used herbs

The most well known herbs are probably garlic and comfrey.

### Garlic

Garlic is one of the oldest herbal remedies; Sanskrit documents its use about 5000 years ago and the Chinese have been using it for more than

3000 years. In 1858 Louis Pasteur demonstrated its anti-bacterial effects and scientific evidence supporting the medicinal uses of garlic has been gaining strength since 1983 when it was revealed that covering the skin of laboratory mice with garlic oil inhibited skin cancer.

Garlic is arguably the best known and most widely used herb in the horse world:

- It is used in respiratory disorders and as an expectorant, it encourages the expulsion of mucus from the lungs.
- As a natural antibiotic.
- It is rich in sulphur, which is excreted through the pores of the skin and helps to deter biting flies.
- As a blood purifier, it is claimed to be helpful for horses prone to laminitis, arthritis, sweet itch and skin problems.
- As an aid to digestion, it supports the development of natural bacterial flora in the gut, while killing pathogens.
- As a preventative against many kinds of infection, it can guard against coughs and viral infections, and also prevent cuts, lacerations and bite wounds from festering.
- As a boost for the immune system, it may be used during and after any course of antibiotics.

Inside the clove there are two substances: alliin and alliinase which have no smell and are separated from each other. When the clove is crushed or sliced the two react to produce sulphur-containing volatile compounds which are thought to be responsible for most of garlic's pharmacological properties. They include: allicin (which gives garlic its characteristic smell), diallyl disulphide, diallyl trisulphide and many others. This means that when allinase acts on alliin to produce allicin, garlic begins to smell like garlic. Allicin is unstable and rapidly reverts to ajoene (pronounced ah-hoe-ene) and dithiins (pronounced di-thigh-eins) or to diallyl disulphide. Levels of allicin can vary widely, even in so-called 'pure' garlic sources, depending on the source of the garlic and how it has been processed. Some forms of processing drive off the beneficial volatile substances, reducing the effectiveness of the product.

*Comfrey*

Comfrey has been used for hundreds of years as a remedy for internal and external ailments. It is said to promote regeneration of bone and body

**Table 9.2**  Which herb to use when.

| Symptom | Herb to use |
| --- | --- |
| Abscess | garlic, echinacea |
| Boil | garlic, echinacea |
| Ulcer | marigold, comfrey |
| Wart | thuja, nettle |
| Eczema | burdock |
| Itching and minor cuts | marigold |
| Cramps | cramp bark, wild yam |
| Infection | arnica |
| Rheumatism | cayenne, ginger |
| Pain | cayenne, ginger |
| Sciatica | St John's wort |
| Bruises and sprains | witch hazel, comfrey, arnica |

tissue and to ease inflammation and pain in joints, tendons and muscles. It can also be used as a poultice to ease swelling and pain. Comfrey contains mucilage, tannins, asparagin, allantoin, alkaloids, vitamin $B_{12}$ and vitamin C. Recent studies have indicated a possibility that in large quantities comfrey may be toxic, so some caution should be exercised in its use.

## Ingredients in herbs

The strange-sounding substances contained within herbs are often well-recognised in conventional medicine; for example the tannin contained in witch hazel and comfrey is an astringent and causes a thin layer to form on wounds or inflamed membranes, so promoting rapid healing. The alkaloids are a group of chemicals including morphine, codeine, caffeine and nicotine; they have potent physiological effects, particularly on the nervous system. Mucilages are the slimy, stringy exudates from many plants; internally they have a healing and soothing action on membranes, and externally the plants make good hot compresses as the mucilage tends to retain heat. Allicin is the volatile oil in garlic that gives it its germicidal properties. There are many other active ingredients within herbs, but remember it is the holistic approach that is vital – balancing the whole body so that it is in harmony and thus less likely to fall prey to sickness and disease. Many horse owners grow comfrey and other herbs to supplement their horse's diet. It is a cheap and simple way to help your horse cope with the stress of modern living – perhaps horse owners could do with some too.

# Nutraceuticals and phytochemicals

An increasing number of the additions to the horse's diet are substances which are claimed to have a natural pharmaceutical effect on the horse's body. These substances fall into two main categories:

- Nutraceuticals; specific chemical compounds found in foods that may prevent disease.
- Phytochemicals; naturally occuring bioactive substances found in plants which are said to prevent disease by interacting with the body's natural healing processes. While vitamins, minerals and other nutrients are essential fuels for the maintenance of health, phytochemicals have been shown to provide additional benefits by triggering the body's natural defence systems and protecting the structures that carry on the metabolic function.

In the past, the phytonutrients found in fruits and vegetables were classified as vitamins: flavonoids were known as vitamin P, cabbage factors (glucosinolates and indoles) were called vitamin U, and ubiquinone was vitamin Q. Tocopherol stayed on the list as vitamin E but vitamin designation was dropped for the other nutrients because specific deficiency symptoms could not be established. Scientists grouped phytonutrients into classes on the basis of similar protective functions as well as individual physical and chemical characteristics of the molecules.

## Terpenes

Terpenes such as those found in green foods, soy products and grains, comprise one of the largest classes of phytonutrients. The most intensely studied terpenes are carotenoids such as beta-carotene. The terpenes function as antioxidants, protecting lipids, blood and other body fluids from assault by free radical oxygen species including singlet oxygen, hydroxyl, peroxide and superoxide radicals.

## Carotenoids

This terpene subclass consists of bright yellow, orange and red plant pigments found in vegetables such as tomatoes, parsley, oranges, pink grapefruit and spinach. There are more than 600 naturally occurring carotenoids, fewer than 10 per cent of which have vitamin A activity. Carotenes also enhance immune response and protect skin cells against UV radiation.

## Limonoids

This terpene subclass, found in citrus fruit peels, appears to be specifically directed to protection of lung tissue.

## Phytosterols

Sterols occur in most plant species. Although green and yellow vegetables contain significant amounts, their seeds concentrate the sterols. Phytosterols compete with dietary cholesterol for uptake in the intestines. They have demonstrated the ability to block the uptake of cholesterol and facilitate its excretion from the body. Other investigations have revealed that phytosterols block the development of tumours in colon, breast and prostate glands.

## Phenols

Phenols protect plants from oxidative damage and perform the same function for humans. Blue, blue-red and violet colorations seen in berries, grapes and aubergine are due to their phenolic content. The outstanding phytonutrient feature of phenols is their ability to block specific enzymes that cause inflammation. They also modify the prostaglandin pathways and thereby protect platelets from clumping.

## Flavonoids

Phytonutrients of this phenol subclass enhance the effects of ascorbate-vitamin C. Flavonoids were once classified as vitamin P, but there are well over 1500 of them, including:

- Flavones (containing the flavonoid apigenin found in chamomile)
- Flavonols (quercetin – grapefruit; rutin – buckwheat; ginkgo-flavonglycosides – ginkgo)
- Flavanones (hesperidin – citrus fruits; silybin – milk thistle).

The biologic activities of flavonoids include action against allergies, inflammation, free radicals, microbes and viruses. Flavonoids also protect the vascular system and strengthen the tiny capillaries that carry oxygen and essential nutrients to all cells.

## Anthocyanidins

This group of flavonoids provides crosslinks that connect and strengthen the intertwined strands of collagen protein. Collagen is the most abundant protein in the body, making up soft tissues, tendons, ligaments and bone matrix. Its great tensile strength depends on preservation of its crosslinks. Anthocyanidins, being water soluble, scavenge free radicals they encounter in tissue fluids. This is a powerful ability especially beneficial for athletes because heavy exercise generates large amounts of free radicals.

### Catechins, gallic acids

The most common catechins are gallic esters, named epicatechin (EC), epicatechin gallate (ECG), and epigallocatechin gallate (EGCG). All are found in green tea, *Camellia sinensis*, and are thought to be responsible for the protective benefits of this beverage.

### Allylic sulphides

Garlic and onions are the most potent members of this thiol subclass, which also includes leeks, shallots and chives. As a group, allylic sulphides appear to possess antimutagenic and anticarcinogenic properties, as well as immune and cardiovascular protection.

### Lipoic acid and ubiquinone

Lipoic acid and ubiquinone (coenzyme Q) are important antioxidants that work to extend the effects of other antioxidants. The roles of both lipoic acid and ubiquinone as antioxidants have been discovered relatively recently. Both have important roles in energy production.

## Probiotics

The horse's gut is populated by bacteria which are essential for the proper digestion of fibre and the health of the horse. These bacteria are susceptible to changes in the horse's gut caused by changes in feeding, strenuous exercise, travelling, irregular feeding and changes in surroundings – in other words stress.

Probiotics can be defined as: 'a live microbial feed supplement which beneficially affects the host animal by improving its intestinal microbial balance'. More simply, probiotics are bacteria which are cultured in laboratory conditions and are then used to redress the balance of the microflora, which has become unbalanced because of stress, illness, or as a result of the use of antibiotics. By re-balancing the microflora the health of the animal can be maintained or substantially improved. Not only does the microflora aid digestion but it also has a major influence on the ability of the host to resist disease and to recover from infections, especially of the digestive tract. Probiotics are used to replenish the naturally occurring beneficial micro-organisms present in the gut and are especially useful at times of stress, including illness, post-operative and antibiotic treatment, travel and exertion.

Probiotics are thought to reduce the effects of stress on the gut micro-organisms in several ways

- By changing the micro-organisms in the gut and reducing the incidence of disease-causing *E. Coli*.
- By stimulating immunity to other bacteria.
- By colonising the digestive tract.
- By producing stimulating substances.
- By reducing toxic substances.

Probiotics are used in agriculture as a natural alternative to hormone implants and in-feed antibiotics. Probiotics are produced from known beneficial bacteria, cultured under strict quality control in the laboratory, preserved to maintain viability and formulated for oral administration. They have been shown to control scouring and improve growth in foals. Probiotics help restore the natural balance of the gut microflora so that the horse can quickly return to its normal nutrition, growth and health status.

Most probiotics fed to horses are a blend of different strains of bacteria. They are protected to survive the acidity of the stomach so that they pass into the intestine, where they colonise. They are presented as pastes to be administered orally or as a compound to be added to the feed.

## Enzymes

Some supplements make use of enzymes: these act as biological catalysts, speeding up cell reactions, without entering the reaction themselves. The breakdown of food into substances small enough to be absorbed across the gut wall is brought about by digestive enzymes. Adding enzymes to the horse's ration is said to have several advantages.

- To increase the digestibility of nutrients which cannot be broken down by naturally occurring enzymes.

- To break down substances in feeds that would otherwise inhibit the digestive process.
- To breakdown specific chemical bonds in feeds that are not degraded by naturally occurring enzymes.
- To aid the breakdown of cellulose.
- To supplement the natural supply of enzymes.

These effects combine to make the feed more digestible, allowing you to feed fewer concentrates or for your horse to put on condition.

Some enzyme preparations are said to bring about a change in the gut micro-organisms in much the same way as a probiotic, improving the health status of the horse and its ability to resist disease.

## Yeast

Another naturally occurring organism that has been beneficially added to horse ration is yeast. The yeast culture is preserved so that it does not lose its viability. When fed to the horse, it passes through the stomach and small intestine to colonise the large intestine, where it stimulates cellulose digesting bacteria, enabling the horse to utilise fibre more efficiently. The yeast appears to stabilise the gut resulting in a better digestive pattern, with less chance of bad behaviour due to minor digestive discomfort. Horses will gain weight with no increase in either hay or concentrates.

Yeasts may also

- produce enzymes
- produce B vitamins
- inhibit growth of 'bad' bugs.

Strains commonly used include, *Saccharomyces cerevisia* and *Aspergillus orizae*.

## Keep blocks

Many horses and ponies are outwintered, being fed hay and concentrates in the field. Feeding concentrates in the field is always fraught with difficulty, with horses fighting and buckets going everywhere. Very often an owner is only able to visit the field once a day, while horses may need feeding night and morning. A practical alternative is a keep block made of cereals, vegetable proteins, minerals and vitamins bound together and fed in a container. This provides a weatherproof self help feed which is easy to use and stops bullying, and together with hay should maintain out-wintered ponies with no further supplementation. Brood mares and youngstock may need further feed, depending on the grass available and the hay quality.

## Supplements for the immune system

### Echinacea

Resembling a black-eyed Susan, echinacea or purple coneflower is a North American perennial. Herbalists consider echinacea one of the best blood purifiers and an effective antibiotic. It activates the body's immune system increasing the chances of fighting off any disease. Since the early 1900s hundreds of scientific articles have been written about echinacea. Most of the research during the past 10 years has focused on the immunostimulant properties of the plant.

The constituents of echinacea include essential oil, polysaccharides, polyacetylenes, betain, glycoside, sesquiterpenes and caryophylene. It also contains copper, iron, tannins, protein, fatty acids and vitamins A, C and E. The most important immune-stimulating components are the large polysaccharides, such as inulin, that increase the production of T-cells and increase other natural killer cell activity. Fat-soluble alkylamides and a caffeic acid glycoside called echinacoside also contribute to the herb's immune empowering effects.

Echinacea it has been shown in animal and human studies to improve the migration of white blood cells to attack foreign micro-organisms and toxins in the bloodstream, implying that it may offer benefit for nearly all infectious conditions. Studies show echinacea prevents the formation of an enzyme which destroys a natural barrier between healthy tissue and damaging organisms.

The antibacterial properties of echinacea can stimulate wound healing and are of benefit to skin conditions; its anti-inflammatory properties may relieve arthritis.

Echinacea products are used as a general nonspecific stimulant to the immune system, supporting and stabilizing cellular immunity and cleansing the blood, for the prevention and treatment of infections. There are no known side effects associated with its use.

### Cat's claw

Cat's claw is a tropical vine that grows in rainforest and jungle areas in South America and Asia. Some cultures refer to the plant as the 'Sacred Herb of the Rainforest'. This vine gets its name from the small thorns at the base of the leaves, which look like a cat's claw. These claws enable the vine to attach itself around trees climbing to heights up to 100 feet.

The plant is considered a valuable medicinal resource and is protected in Peru. Although scientific research has just recently begun to explore cat's claw, many cultures native to the South American rainforest areas have used this herb for hundreds of years.

The active substances in cat's claw are alkaloids, tannins and several other phytochemicals. Some of the alkaloids have been proven to boost the immune system. By stimulating the immune system, it can also improve response to viral and respiratory infections. The major alkaloid, rhynchophylline, has anti-hypertensive effects while other constituents contribute anti-inflammatory, antioxidant and anti-cancer properties.

### Aloe vera

*Aloe vera* is an exceptional healing plant with an extensive history of use. Researchers have found that fresh aloe gel promotes wound healing by speeding up the growth of skin cells and aiding recovery from surgery. Aloe has also proved effective in treating pressure sores, chronic leg ulcers, and frostbite. *Aloe vera* has also been shown to have strong anti-bacterial and antifungal properties against a broad range of microbes. Carrisyn, an extract of aloe, has shown recent evidence of being able to inhibit a number of viruses *in vitro*. Carrisyn appears to work by stimulating the immune system to trigger the production of T cells, thereby increasing immune function. Other active ingredients of the aloe plant include 'salicylates', which control inflammation and pain, and an enzyme that inhibits 'bradykinin', the chemical messenger responsible for transmitting pain signals through the nerves. Aloe also contains 'magnesium lactate', a chemical known to inhibit the release of histamines responsible for skin irritation and itching:

## Supplements for soundness

### Glucosamine hydrochloride and chondroitin sulphate

Glucosamine hydrochloride and chondroitin sulphate are known as chondroprotective agents along with the antioxidant vitamins and methylsulphonylmethane (MSM). Due to the weight-bearing and mechanical functions of the joints, the connective tissue matrix (namely collagen and proteoglycans) is under constant rebuilding. Chondroprotective agents support or enhance the connective tissue matrix and the synthesis of joint fluid, and inhibit degeneration and inflammation of joints and soft tissue. These substances have key roles in the function of connective tissue and joints, including:

- building blocks and key precursors of connective tissue
- build and support collagen, hence cartilage
- synthesis of joint fluid
- retention of moisture.

These functions combine to help:

- reduce joint pain
- improve joint function
- and possibly inhibit joint degeneration.

*Glucosamine hydrochloride*

Glucosamine is the key precursor of the synthesis of the connective tissue matrix; it also composes over half of hyaluronic acid found in the joint structures. Being key in the rate-limiting step, glucosamine stimulates production of glycosaminoglycans (GAGs), like hyaluronic acid and chondroitin sulphate, fundamental in the production of collagen and finally, connective tissue. In recent human and dog trials, glucosamine supplementation showed significant reduction of joint pain, tenderness and swelling, and improved joint function in a short period of time.

*Vitamin C*

Vitamin C is involved in a number of biochemical processes. Most importantly the body needs vitamin C to grow, maintain, and repair structural tissues. Vitamin C has been shown to have an integral role in the production of specific proteins, like collagen, and other structural elements of connective tissues. The antioxidative qualities of vitamin C also limit the deterioration of connective tissues by free radicals; these are highly-reactive, oxygen-containing chemicals which can damage equine cells and tissues, including cartilage. The antioxidant vitamins C, E and beta-carotene neutralise free radicals and other reactive chemicals and help protect the body's cells.

## Chondroitin sulphate

Chondroitin sulphate is a mucopolysaccharide which helps to form the cartilage matrix. As a nutritional supplement, this naturally occurring compound provides support for strong, healthy cartilage and joints.

Bovine cartilage contains significant proportions of proteoglycans, integral substances for building and maintaining the ground substances of cartilage. It provides a safe and natural way to support healthy joints, through its ability to build up cartilage.

Shark cartilage is renowned for providing potent support for the maintenance of healthy joints and cartilage. It is a natural source of proteoglycans. In particular, shark cartilage contains chondroitin sulphate, one of the most potent proteoglycans known. There is debate about the ethics of feeding horses shark and bovine cartilage as a source of chondroitin sulphate.

## MSM (methylsulphonylmethane)

MSM is a source of organic sulphur, an essential component of connective tissue, skin, hooves, amino acids. It is said to:

- reduce inflammation
- improve joint mobility
- maintain the integrity of lung tissue.

Pure MSM is one of the most bioavailable sources of sulphur. Sulphur from MSM is used in the formation of numerous protein-rich structures in the body. MSM contributes sulphur to the disulphide bonds that are essential for the proper conformation of hair, horn and connective tissue proteins. Even hormones and antibodies receive sulphur from MSM. Like vitamin $B_{12}$, methionine, and dimethylglycine (DMG), MSM is a methyl donor nutrient; the body can use methyl units from these nutrients to increase the flexibility and capacity of its biochemistry.

It has been suggested that MSM could have many useful applications for horses including:

- Improvement of osteoarthritic conditions.
- Reduction of lung dysfunction.
- Moderation of allergic responses.

- Control of hyperacidity – many performance horses are thought to suffer from some degree of acid-induced ulcerations as a result of high carbohydrate diets. MSM appears to bind with the mucous membranes, creating a paint-like coating.
- Regulation of immune function.

## Supplements for performance

### Free radicals and antioxidants

Free radicals are highly damaging electrically charged compounds of oxygen, such as superoxide radical ($O_2^-$), hydroxy radical ($OH^-$) and hydrogen peroxide ($H_2O_2$). Free radicals are capable of damaging biochemical compounds and affecting cell activities; they are produced as natural by-products of normal metabolic function. This means that essential chemicals present in the horse's body can contribute to the development of diseases such as arthritis and post-viral syndrome. Intense exertion, stress, disease, trauma and injury all lead to oxidative stress, i.e. the production of free radicals. Free radicals are neutralised by antioxidants (free radical scavengers). These include:

- vitamins C, E and beta-carotene (precursor of vitamin A)
- trace minerals Se, Zn, Cu
- polyphenol groups, e.g. flavonoids.

### Flavonoids

Flavonoids possess anti-inflammatory, anti-allergic, anti-microbial and anti-viral properties. Flavonoids were once classified as vitamin P, but there are well over 1500 of them, including:

- Flavones (containing the flavonoid apigenin found in chamomile).
- Flavonols (quercetin – grapefruit; rutin – buckwheat; ginkgo-flavonglycosides – ginkgo).
- Flavanones (hesperidin – citrus fruits; silybin – milk thistle).

### Vitamin E and selenium

Vitamin E is an antioxidant that prevents premature reaction of oxygen in the body, thus preventing the breakdown of many substances in the body. It is essential to the use of oxygen by muscles, helps improve circulation, promotes normal clotting and healing and prolongs the life of red blood cells. It acts as an antioxidant to help protect cells from free radical injury and is key for normal growth and development. Selenium is also an important antioxidant preventing the formation of free radicals. Along with Vitamin E, it aids in normal body growth and fertility.

## Chromium

Chromium helps in carbohydrate utilisation and is involved in metabolism of glucose (for energy). It is an essential co-factor for insulin function in the body. Insulin is released whenever carbohydrate is digested, its purpose is to control the body's level of blood sugar and convert extra sugar into stored energy. When the body releases insulin, it also releases chromium into the blood stream in order to facilitate insulin in its action. Chromium is also involved in the synthesis of fatty acids and cholesterol and it also helps bring protein to where it is needed.

# Appendix 1
# Units and Formulations

## Units

The daily requirements of horses and ponies, necessary to keep them alive, healthy and able to undertake various levels of performance, are estimated in terms of the amounts of each essential nutrient required per day. These essential nutrients come under the main headings of energy, minerals, trace elements, vitamins and protein, the last being made up of amino acids such as lysine and methionine.

It is very important to consider the total daily feed intake – all the feed eaten by the horse during the day and, when considering individual requirements, the total daily intake of each – what the horse actually takes in. As an example, a horse may obtain the same satisfactory protein intake from a high protein hard feed plus a low protein forage as he does from a low protein hard feed plus a high protein forage. In feed analysis, each of the nutrients is commonly measured and quoted in particular units, and it is useful to know what they are and what they mean when applied to the total daily feed intake of a horse.

The following is a brief explanation of each.

*Kilogram (kg) and pound (lb)*

The common weight measurements used for feeds, forages and raw materials. Quite simply:

1 kg = 2.205 lb
1 lb = 0.454 kg
1000 kg = 1 tonne

*Gram (g), milligram (mg), microgram (mcg) and ounce (oz)*

Used for the nutrients present in smaller quantities by weight.

1 oz = 28.35 g
1 g = 0.035 oz
1 g = 1000 mg
1 mg = 1000 mcg

## Grams per kilogram (g/kg)

This means the number of grams of the nutrient in each kilogram of the whole sample. For example, oats may contain 0.7 g/kg calcium, which means that each kilogram (or 2.205 lb) contains 0.7 grams of the mineral calcium.

Similarly mg/kg refers to the number of milligrams contained in one kilogram, and mcg/kg, the number of micrograms in a kilogram.

## Percentage

This shows the nutrient expressed as part of 100, so if the protein percentage given for a feed is 10 per cent, it means that in each 100 kg of the feed there are 10 kg of protein, and in each 100 lb of feed there are 10 lb of protein.

## Energy

Energy is usually described as Metabolisable Energy (ME) or Digestible Energy (DE). A simple explanation of these terms is:

Total or Gross Energy in a feed, less the energy lost in the faeces resulting from eating that feed, leaves
The Digestible Energy (DE) in the feed; less the energy lost in the urine excreted and the waste gases produced from eating that feed, leaves
The Metabolisable Energy (ME).

Energy is usually measured as kilocalories per kilogram (kcal/kg) or megajoules per kilogram (MJ/kg), and the relationship between these is 1MJ = 239.23 kcal. Joules are metric calories.

## International units

The unit of measurement used for vitamins A, D and E. An approximate relationship on a weight basis is:

1 iu of vitamin A = 0.3 micrograms
1 iu of vitamin D = 0.025 micrograms
1 iu of vitamin E = 1 milligram

*Dry matter/as fed*

In all instances the analysis of a feed material may be shown on a Dry Matter (DM) basis, which means that calculations are made after the exclusion of any moisture content in the material. Analysis may be on an 'as fed' (AF) basis, which either means that the calculation takes into account the moisture content of the feed, or assumes a level moisture content, usually of 10 per cent or 12 per cent (90 per cent or 88 per cent dry matter). A calculation made on dry matter always gives a higher figure than one on an 'as fed' basis, and is a more accurate measurement for comparisons between feeds and feed materials.

## Formulation

The practical formulation of a daily ration for a horse or pony means taking the feed materials available and calculating how much of each, on a weight basis, should be fed in order to supply the horse with its daily requirement of nutrients.

Firstly, it is necessary to have an idea of how much of each nutrient is required. There are some 'rules of thumb' that help for adult horses:

(1)  The total daily feed intake should not be much higher than 2.5 per cent of the horse's liveweight or the horse may have difficulty consuming the full quantity.

(2)  The roughage or fibrous portion of the diet should not be much lower than 0.5 per cent of the horse's liveweight in most circumstances.

(3)  The daily protein intake should be between about 700 g and 1500 g per day, which means that if a horse is eating 11 kg (24 lb) total feed per day, the average daily feed protein should be about 6.5 to 13.5 per cent.

(4)  The minimum daily calcium intake should be about 25 g per day and the minimum daily phosphorus intake should be about 18 g per day. It is particularly important that the total daily ration always contains more calcium than phosphorus.

(5)  The minimum sodium intake should be about 3 g/kg of ration, and

diets containing 5–10 g/kg of common salt will meet normal sodium requirements.

(6) The approximate energy requirements are usually divided into two: firstly, the energy the horse needs for keeping fit and warm, which varies with the liveweight of the horse, and is termed the maintenance energy; secondly, the feed energy needed for work.

*Maintenance energy*

| Bodyweight (kg) | DE required/day (MJ/kg DM) |
|-----------------|----------------------------|
| 430 | 55 |
| 530 | 65 |
| 660 | 75 |

*Exercise: DE required for work above maintenance*

| 1 hour duration of each activity | DE in kcal/kg liveweight |
|----------------------------------|--------------------------|
| Walking | 0.5 |
| Slow trotting, some cantering | 9.0 |
| Fast trot, cantering, some jumping | 17.0 |
| Cantering, galloping, jumping | 30.0 |

Having looked at the basic requirements, it is possible to apply these to an example of a daily ration.

Subject:          Adult horse
                  530 kg liveweight
                  Maintenance + 1 hour fast trotting

Daily ration example:  6.0 kg hay
                  4.5 kg oats
                  1.5 kg sugar beet pulp
                  1.0 kg bran
                  85 g salt
                  56 g limestone flour
                  100 g vitamins/trace elements

The contribution of each nutrient provided by this daily ration can then be calculated. For example, the protein content of each item in the ration is:

| Hay | 7 per cent | × | 6.0 kg | = | 420 g |
|---|---|---|---|---|---|
| Oats | 10 per cent | × | 4.5 kg | = | 450 g |
| Sugar beet pulp | 7 per cent | × | 1.5 kg | = | 105 g |
| Bran | 15 per cent | × | 1.0 kg | = | 150 g |
| Total | | | | = | 1125 g |

Multiplying the percentage protein in each feed material by the amount by weight in the daily ration gives a total protein contribution of 1125 g (8.7 per cent protein in the ration).

The same calculation can be made for each of the nutrients:

*Daily intake calculation*

|  | From ration | Requirement |
|---|---|---|
| Total feed | 13.24 kg | 13.25 kg max |
| Roughage | 6.0 kg | at least 2.65 kg |
| Energy | 123 MJ | at least 103 MJ |
| Protein | 1125 g | at least 700 g |
| Sodium | 50 g | at least 39 g (3 g/kg) |
| Calcium | 55 g | at least 25 g |
| Phosphorus | 39 g | at least 18 g |
| Calcium:phosphorus | 1.4:1.0 | at least 1.1:1.0 |

Vitamins and trace elements are added at the correct level by including 100 g of a reputable vitamin/mineral supplement. If the weather is warm or the horse sweats a lot, extra salt should be added or access to a salt lick should be allowed.

If all the factors noted are taken into account when deciding on the suitability of a daily ration, the horse will be given every possible chance of being extremely fit and healthy.

*Height*

1 hand = 4 inches = 10.16 cm

| Height (hh) | Height (cm) |
|---|---|
| 9 | 91.4 |
| 10 | 101.6 |
| 11 | 111.6 |
| 12 | 121.8 |
| 13 | 132.0 |
| 14 | 142.2 |
| 15 | 152.4 |
| 16 | 162.6 |
| 17 | 172.7 |

# Appendix 2
# Feed Preparation

### Bran mash

(1) Use clean bucket.

(2) Add required amount of bran, usually about 1.5 kg (3.5 lb) plus a teaspoon of salt and a sprinkling of oats if the horse needs to be tempted to eat the mash.

(3) Pour on as much boiling water as the bran will absorb.

(4) Stir well.

(5) Cover to retain the steam and leave to stand until cool.

(6) Before feeding stir in a heaped teaspoon of limestone flour.

Correctly made the mash should have a crumbly texture. Molasses or cooked linseed can be added to make the mash more appetising. A bran mash can be fed the night before a rest day, or after hard work, to tired horses.

### Linseed jelly

(1) Cover linseed with water and soak for 24 hours. Allow 0.5 kg (about 1 lb) linseed per horse.

(2) Add more water and bring to the boil.

(3) Boil for 1–2 hours until the linseed is soft, taking care that the linseed does not stick and burn.

(4) Allow to cool and add the resulting jelly to the horse's feed.

### Linseed tea/mash

(1) Follow the above procedure but use more water so that a tea is formed.

(2) To make a linseed mash, add 1 kg (2 lb) of bran to soak up the fluid, cover until cool.

(3) Feed as a mash.

### Boiled barley

(1) Soak barley for 12 hours.

(2) Boil gently until the grains are just beginning to split and the water has been absorbed.

(3) Add to every feed if horse is lacking condition or add to small feed for a tired horse.

### Gruel

(1) Place 0.5–1 kg (1–2 lb) of oatmeal in a bucket. Add a little cold water and stir to stop the gruel becoming lumpy.

(2) Pour 4–6 litres (1–1.5 gallons) of hot but not boiling water and stir.

(3) Leave to cool.

(4) The tea should be thin enough to drink and is palatable and refreshing to a tired horse.

# Index

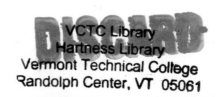